THE
CHOICE

THE
CHOICE

The Abortion Divide in America

DANIELLE D'SOUZA GILL

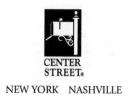

CENTER
STREET®

NEW YORK   NASHVILLE

Center Street
Hachette Book Group
1290 Avenue of the Americas, New York, NY 10104
centerstreet.com
twitter.com/centerstreet

First edition: October 2020

Center Street is a division of Hachette Book Group, Inc. The Center Street name and logo are trademarks of Hachette Book Group, Inc.

The publisher is not responsible for websites (or their content) that are not owned by the publisher.

Library of Congress Cataloging-in-Publication Data has been applied for.

ISBNs: 978-1-5460-9986-4 (hardcover), 978-1-5460-9985-7 (ebook)

Printed in the United States of America

LSC-C

10 9 8 7 6 5 4 3 2 1

For my Dad
Who taught me the most important things in life.

ACKNOWLEDGMENTS

I would like to start by thanking Hachette Book Group, particularly Center Street, for publishing this book. I would like to thank my editor, Kate Hartson, as well as Hentry Hurt, who gave me thoughtful, appreciated criticism. I would like to thank the people who allowed me to interview them in the process of researching this book. Though you remain nameless, I learned a great deal from your expertise, testimony, and insight. I would also like to thank Judi Gill, Hurley Gill, Michelle Knesbach, and Bruce Schooley for reading drafts of this book and offering their time. I would not be where I am today were it not for the scholars I learned from including Donald E. Pease, Lucas A. Swaine, David P. Lagomarsino, and Jonathan V. Crewe. I would also like to thank Robert Mulgrew and Adam Ruderman. I will always be grateful to Lara Trump, Kellyanne Conway, and Kimberly Guilfoyle who believed in me. I would also like to thank Father Michael Jones, Eric Metaxas, Don and Dori Willeman, Father Frank Pavone, Alveda King, the Falwell family, Cardinal Dolan, Abby Johnson, and Carol Swain for their guidance. My husband Brandon is my rock, a constant source of love and encouragement. To my loyal friends and followers on social media, you have seen me grow up and go through formative times in my life. I know

ACKNOWLEDGMENTS

many of you have joined me on what I hope is the beginning of a long journey fighting for truth. I would like to thank the pro-life movement—those who came before me, and those who will come after me. There are many who have been fighting for decades for the pro-life cause and their efforts should never be forgotten. To everyone who feels unnoticed, I want you to know that every prayer prayed for the unborn, every woman whose mind was changed, and every child you saved, matters. And to those to come, the future activists not yet born, I hope you fearlessly carry the pro-life torch.

CONTENTS

CONTENTS

> "Men occasionally stumble over the truth, but most of them pick themselves up and hurry off as if nothing ever happened."
>
> —WINSTON CHURCHILL

Abortion is the great, unexamined issue of our time. When we look at the controversies swirling in America, we see that underneath them lurks this issue of abortion, which is the driving force of what is going on, even when it is not mentioned.

In the Trump presidency, we have seen a succession of controversies from the Mueller Report to Ukraine to Kavanaugh to impeachment to coronavirus. Trump, himself, has been under constant siege since he won in 2016. Most of these controversies had a subtext that went largely unnoticed. On the face of it, the Kavanaugh hearings were about the Me Too movement—women accusing Kavanaugh of having assaulted them or taken advantage of them. There was a fake element to this. One of the women admitted that she was lying and made it up because she wanted to get rid of Kavanaugh. She claimed she was "angry" because of what he represented and wanted her sexual assault allegation to "grab attention."[1]

But why did she want to get rid of Kavanaugh? Because Kavanaugh represented a very real threat to something very important to her, namely, abortion. Many pro-choicers realized that if confirmed, Kavanaugh might be the swing vote in overturning *Roe v. Wade*. When you begin to look under the surface you find that this accuser was motivated by the same thing his other accusers were motivated by. Debra Katz, the lawyer for Kavanaugh's primary accuser, Christine Blasey Ford, said in a speech that *Roe v. Wade* "is part of what motivated Christine."[2] Katz said, "We were going to have a conservative [justice]...Elections have consequences, but he will always have an asterisk next to his name. When he takes a scalpel to *Roe v. Wade*, we will know who he is."[3] The Kavanaugh confirmation that became a show trial was ultimately about abortion.

When we turn to immigration, impeachment, even coronavirus, we see that the Left's focus is on blasting Trump. So what is it about Trump that causes so much apoplexy? Trump was instrumental in bringing about some of the lowest unemployment rates the country has seen in decades. And when coronavirus hit, very early on, Trump was prescient in restricting travel from China, saving innumerable American lives. The same goes for bringing jobs back to America. People quickly realized in the wake of coronavirus that relying so heavily on China has negative effects, especially during a pandemic. Under President Trump, we have even seen ISIS weakened in the Middle East and the death of one of the most powerful terrorists, Qasem Soleimani. So one would think that Trump would receive some credit for this. But, no. Why?

One of the most, if the not the most, threatening things about him is the fact that he is transforming the courts. Not only is he populating the appellate courts with one constitutionalist justice after another, a systematic overhaul of the judiciary, but he is also reshaping the Supreme Court with the Gorsuch and Kavanaugh confirmations. If Trump is reelected, then over the next four years there is a very good chance that the Supreme Court could move to a 6–3 majority, even a 7–2 majority. It was a 7–2 majority that decided *Roe v. Wade*, so it may take a 7–2 majority to overturn it. Supreme Court justices are appointed for life, which is to say that this would be a majority that would long outlast Trump's time in office.

So, from the point of view of the pro-choice Left, Trump signifies a reconstructed Supreme Court—and even a reconstructed America. The Supreme Court can produce lasting changes in American society. Of course, court decisions affect a range of areas, but the single most important issue that the Left is concerned about, the single issue on which the court can have a decisive and momentous impact, is abortion. At the end of the day, the Left's vehement hatred of Trump is rooted in his ability to move the courts in a pro-life direction.

But why does the Left care so much about abortion? Because abortion is at the center of the values the Left has been trying to impose on the culture for the last fifty years. This is the central issue, now at risk, that is driving the Left berserk. Abortion is also a key issue for the Right. Pro-life activists have been fighting since before 1973, and they are not giving up anytime soon.

What makes this phenomenon so interesting is that abortion, while being at the center of American politics, is at the same time rarely openly debated in a fundamental way. This is not to say that there aren't skirmishes about abortion when a heartbeat bill is introduced or that there isn't an ongoing Twitter battle about it. These are episodic instances in which people talk about abortion, take a stance on abortion, and speak about the extremities of abortion, but those on the Left are almost never willing to debate a pro-life person. They won't do it, you'll notice. Almost anyone prominent on the Left, even when this is their "main issue," will almost always decline. They imply that there's not a whole lot else to say about this issue. The Supreme Court settled the abortion issue in 1973, and it has remained that way for the last fifty years. Therefore, the debate is today pretty much the same as it was then, so there's nothing new to say.

Nothing could be further from the truth. The world today is completely different than it was fifty years ago. We are not living in the atmosphere of *Roe v. Wade*. Even the key terms of the debate have changed dramatically. One of the crucial concepts used by the Supreme Court in discussing abortion was the issue of viability, which refers to the ability of the unborn fetus to live outside the womb. For the court, viability determined the point at which states could, in theory, restrict abortion, even though in practice, *Roe v. Wade* permitted very little such regulation. Before viability, states were permitted no restriction whatsoever. The concept of viability was a critical criterion for the court that decided *Roe*.

Yet, if we look at viability, we see that the moment that an unborn fetus can exist outside the womb has moved earlier and earlier. Viability will likely continue to move earlier as technology advances, and no one can predict how early it will become. The basis of the Supreme Court's decision has been swept away by advancements in technology.

The Supreme Court in *Roe v. Wade* also insisted that there was a great cloud of uncertainty over whether the fetus is a human life, a person. In fact, the court excavated details from history, including ancient history, that suggest there was a great deal of confusion about the process of coming into being. And the court even affirmed the notion that it might ultimately be a dogmatic or religious question as to when life begins. This was a philosophical matter, the court implied, that ultimately reasonable people could disagree upon and perhaps each person could take their own position on. Once again, this agnostic view has been seriously called into question if not completely invalidated by modern science. I explain this in detail in the first section of the book.

And in the case of fetal development, we are not just referring to medical opinion, we're referring to modern science, which enables us to observe life with the naked eye. The development of the fetus itself can now be directly observed inside the womb thanks to the technology of ultrasound. One can see the development of the unborn. Very early on, we easily see a recognizable human being in the process of growing, moving, and responding. This is not merely a supposition. It is a direct observation.

Rarely do we see an abortion debate, a genuine discussion, an engagement with the arguments, so that is what I am going to do in this book. Far from being settled, the abortion debate is coming back to life in full force as both sides muster their forces. There's a new generation of young people who are looking at it with fresh eyes. And I am a member of this generation. I am a young woman in my twenties who can see that this is the crucial moral issue of our time, very much in the way that slavery was the crucial moral issue of the nineteenth century. I explore this in detail in several chapters but will only touch on it here.

As with slavery, the anxiety that surrounded Abraham Lincoln, in the critical year of 1860, focused on that one issue. There were other issues swirling about—including tariffs and the relative economic power of the North and the South—and some think that it was those issues that actually drove the war. But, no. What drove the war was Lincoln's election. And why was Lincoln's election so frightening?

Alexander Stephens, a Democrat who later became the vice president of the Confederacy, did not initially want to secede from the Union. Prior to secession, he gave a speech at a secession convention in Georgia. Stephens urged his fellow Georgians not to break from the Union. His argument was simple. Abraham Lincoln can't do very much. Sure, he has been elected, but the Democrats still control the Senate. Lincoln does not have a decisive majority in the House. And so Stephens's point is: we can block him. We can prevent him from doing any harm to the institution of slavery. We can have slavery and Lincoln at the same time.[4]

But, of course, the South didn't go along with Stephens on this. Why? The South was terrified that Lincoln's election represented a tipping point. If new territories and new states came into the Union as free states, not slave states, the population and number of free states would continue to increase, while the number of slave states remained the same. This meant that the free states would become a permanent majority, and at some future time, they could even be so numerous, and their power in the electoral college so strong, that they could amend the Constitution to end slavery. The South knew that prospect might be somewhat distant. But Southerners saw themselves as stronger at that point than they would be in the future, and they knew their position would erode further and further. Now was the time, they resolved, to strike a blow, or else all would be lost.

Something very similar is going on with the pro-choice Left

today. There is a deep anxiety that Trump's election and reelection represent a threat to abortion "rights," and to the Court, that might prove irreversible, at least for the foreseeable future. The pro-choice Left doesn't even hesitate to threaten the Supreme Court. In a remarkable statement without precedent, Senate Minority Leader Chuck Schumer (D-NY) issued a warning. On March 3, 2020, the eve of a Supreme Court decision relating to abortion, he stood in front of a crowd on the steps outside the court and declared, "I want to tell you, Gorsuch. I want to tell you, Kavanaugh: You have unleashed the whirlwind, and you will pay the price."[5] Schumer warned, "You won't know what hit you if you go forward with these awful decisions."[6]

In a rare rebuke, Chief Justice John Roberts replied, "Threatening statements of this sort from the highest levels of government are not only inappropriate, they are dangerous. All members of the Court will continue to do their job, without fear or favor, from whatever quarter."[7]

In 2019, New York passed a bill stating that a woman can get an abortion at nine months, removing any meaningful restrictions on late-term abortions. The Democrats in New York couldn't wait to pass this bill; meanwhile every Republican in New York's State Senate voted against it. Democratic Governor Andrew Cuomo signed the bill into law, stating the bill was an "historic victory for New Yorkers and our progressive values."[8] On January 22, 2019, New York City lit up the Freedom Tower pink to celebrate this momentous occasion. Cuomo said that the pink light would "celebrate this achievement, and shine a bright light forward for the rest of the nation to follow."[9]

It is not a statement of insult, but merely of fact, to note that the pro-abortion Left has become a champion of mass killing. Abortion is a form of mass killing. It is going on in America and in other countries in the twenty-first century.

Mass killing used to be a part of life for humans, but the world has developed and progressed since then, on every level. We have developed an aversion to holocaust and to genocide. Individual cases of suffering are abhorrent. There are environmental tragedies that cause chaos. But in general, as a species, we try to eliminate human suffering that occurs on a mass scale, particularly suffering that is inflicted on humans by other humans. And yet there is precisely such a form of suffering, in fact of killing, going on—the killing of the unborn. But normal people in society, for the most part, are blind to it. Many people are indifferent to it, seem not to care, and instead worry more about other things, trivial things in comparison with this important thing.

Abortion is the greatest form of mass killing in the world by far. Abortion kills more people than war, famine, and genocide combined. In 2018, HIV/AIDS took 1.7 million lives, cancer took 8.2 million, and abortion took 41.9 million lives.[10] And that's in 2018 alone. This is a worldwide tragedy. But we happen to be the worst offenders in the United States. We have an abortion industry, one might almost say a factory of mass killing. Its name is Planned Parenthood.

Incredibly, in many people's minds this is a reputable organization, worthy of one's charitable donations. This is an organization perceived to be doing good in the world. One could almost think of the concentration camps in Germany and in the occupied territories constructing themselves as nonprofit institutions, running ads on TV, portraying themselves in a benign light, and asking the German people to contribute money for the operations of death occurring within those institutions. It's creepy, and it demands investigation and explanation.

How in modern America, a society with so much wealth, a society that proclaims loudly the virtue of compassion, can we support the killing of the disadvantaged and the voiceless in our midst? Abortion is the dark side of America. It is so dark that it is enough to call into question the American dream, the American experiment, the goodness of America. It is enough to shake one's patriotism and force us to reexamine our country, the principles it's based on, our consciences, and what we believe in. The reason is not merely the widespread practice of abortion in America but also the fact that America has the most radical pro-abortion policies in the world. Abortion in our country is legalized by the Supreme Court. It is affirmed by governmental institutions. It is practiced and publicized by nonprofit institutions. It is ingrained in the medical profession. It is normalized in practice in society. Many people do it. Many people think it's acceptable. Some people even think it's a positive good.

In this respect, one could compare abortion to the practice of slavery in the American South. Slavery was a practice that was at the root of the Southern economy, a practice that was sustained in laws, supported by the states, and then routinized in the practice of plantations not merely the cotton plantations, but also rice plantations, tobacco plantations and then even in urban areas, where domestic slaves worked as apprentices for carpenters, masons, and other professionals. Here, too, abortion is sustained by an elaborate legal infrastructure and an abortion industry that operates very profitably across the country. In America, abortion is "on demand."

In not just New York but seven states, it is legal to get an abortion throughout your nine months of pregnancy, even when you are dilating and about to go into labor. According to Governor Ralph Northam of Virginia, it should be possible to continue an abortion even after a baby is born. In other words, if you attempt an abortion, it fails, the baby turns up on the doctor's table, it could then be made comfortable and left to die. To me, this is infanticide and by itself represents a disturbing shift in the abortion debate. It was only a couple of decades ago under Bill Clinton that we heard that abortion should be "safe, legal, and rare." We don't even hear that language coming from the Left anymore. It's almost as if abortion now is promoted as something that should be safe, legal, celebrated, and commonplace.

Most of the industrialized world permits abortion in some fashion but keeps it regulated. In many European countries, as well as Australia and Canada, abortion is permitted in the early stages of pregnancy, restricted in the middle stages of pregnancy, and outlawed in the late stages of pregnancy, except in extreme circumstances, such as when the mother's life or health is seriously endangered.

In America, however, this approach to abortion does not exist. Not only has abortion been allowed, but even attempted restrictions on abortion that are very minor, often aimed not at protecting unborn life but at protecting just the woman's health, are struck down. The pro-choice Left wants abortion to be available everywhere, at any time, and to be free, which is to say they want the government to subsidize abortion for people who can't afford one. There are many organizations promoting abortion, and Shout Your Abortion is one of them. Celebrities like Oprah have promoted this effort, which encourages women to own and embrace abortion as a form of feminine identity.[11]

Here, again, the analogy to slavery is illuminating. Initially, during the time of the American founding, slavery was seen as a bad thing. Even Thomas Jefferson, for example, who owned two hundred slaves, denounced slavery, sometimes in the cadence of a biblical prophet. Jefferson spoke of the elimination of slavery as the shared moral aspiration of the American colonies. Never once did he defend it as a good thing. He didn't know what to do about it. In a letter to John Holmes, Jefferson wrote of slavery, "We have the wolf by the ear, and we can neither hold him, nor safely let him go."[12] And that was, in general, the attitude toward abortion in the late part of the twentieth century. Abortion was seen as a necessary evil but not as a positive good.

In the nineteenth century, an aggressive pro-slavery campaign developed in the American South, with some supporters in the North, that affirmed slavery. They said that slavery was good not only for the slave owner but also for the slave. This is called the positive good school of slavery, and this is exactly what we've seen emerging with abortion—abortion as a positive good. Abortion is good not only for the mother but also for the unborn. You'll hear proponents say: Some people are better off dead. Some people will have better lives if they don't have lives at all than if they have lives that are seen as not worth living. I discuss these utilitarian arguments in the latter part of the book.

Let's remember that abortion as a form of mass killing is avoidable. This is a mass killing that we have accepted and even adopted in this country. Meanwhile, there are deaths that occur around the world due to circumstances that seem outside human control. Children in other countries die due to famine, malnutrition, and disease because their families and communities don't have the resources to save them. There are not enough doctors around, and the governments are helpless. But that is completely different than what's happening in America, where we have enough resources, we have enough doctors to birth babies, and the unborn are purposefully and intentionally killed, even though there is the infrastructure, there is modern medicine, there are the hospitals, and there are families on long waiting lists to adopt. This is a country with a high life expectancy, perhaps the richest country in the world, and yet mass killing is going on here.

How can it be going on? Why is it going on? How can America, a country devoted to the right to life, liberty, and the pursuit of happiness, let this go on? How can we allow the normalization of mass killing? In Nazi Germany, the Jews and other war captives were considered "the other." They were portrayed as the stranger, the outsider, or the alien. In the case of abortion, however, the tragedy doesn't involve a mother killing any child but a mother killing her own child. The child shares half of her DNA. How can this happen in modern society?

Historically, if we look back at the ancient world, we do find cases of parents killing their own children. In some cases, in ancient Sparta, for example, families would leave their baby in the cold on a hillside to find it dead in the morning. In Sparta, the justification for this practice was the belief that the child was weak and unfit for the harsh routines of Spartan society. Today, we look upon that practice, correctly, as a form of barbarism. In other societies where we find infants murdered by their parents, it is typically only in desperate circumstances, as when the smothering of a baby was intended to save the lives of the other children because the family would otherwise be discovered and killed or when the parents did not have enough food to feed the children they already had, and a new one coming along would be sure to die from starvation.

In very dire circumstances, this does happen. But normally, it is very hard for parents to kill their offspring. Mothers instinctively throw themselves in front of a car or a bus to push their child out of the way. Parents, especially mothers, are biologically programmed to love their children. In many ways the child in the womb is more attached to the mother at that point than any point in the future, with the mother able to feel the child kick and move and with both sharing food and nutrients.

So we have to ask, in an honest way, how did mass killing become normalized? The answer is twofold. First, there is a denial that killing is going on. Abortion clinics like Planned Parenthood know the power of denial, and they exploit it. Planned Parenthood, for example, doesn't like to show the sonogram to a woman seeking an abortion. Why? Because they know that if the woman sees her child in the womb, she will likely walk out of the clinic.

Abortionists routinely operate by using deception. While the abortionist can hear the baby's heartbeat go from a beating pulse to silence, the woman does not; the woman is left in the dark. The abortionist can see the baby's gender, but the woman does not. The abortionist can see the baby in the womb literally move away from the lethal injection and try to get away from it, trying to save its life, but the woman doesn't see those movements. Women are purposely led through the abortion process so that they remain in denial, and only later in life, after the procedure and upon reflection, do many women realize the loss of the child that would have been their own son or daughter.

Even a woman's decision to have an abortion, when she could put the baby up for adoption, shows the power of denial. Why? Because aborting the child somehow makes you believe that the child has gone away. Then you can go on with your life as if it never existed. Alternatively, once the child is born, you see it. It's harder to ignore. Even if you give it up for adoption immediately, and it remains a closed adoption where identities are not disclosed, the child is still somewhere out there in this world. There's a child walking around who looks like you, has 50 percent of your genes, is related to you, and was birthed by you. Somebody else who loves the child is raising that child, but this can still be a disturbing thought to a mother. But I ask, if this is disturbing, why is killing the child any less disturbing?

Many horrific things go on in the world, and we often don't do anything about them because we can't see them. In some cases, we don't want to see them. For example, we know in the abstract that there are underage children working in factories in China. They're making some of our clothes and our iPhones, which we happily use. Our shoes are made in sweatshops, and we still buy them. It is a fact that we don't like to see people suffer, and don't like to think about it either, so we would rather look the other way and act like it's not happening.

This is the same reason that the Nazis put the death camps outside Germany. The death camps were all in occupied territory, with most of them in Poland. The Nazis wanted to shield the German public from the gruesome reality of the Final Solution. Even if people in Germany knew that there were terrible things going on, the Nazis didn't want them to see those things because then their consciences might revolt. And so the Nazis relied, one may say, on mass denial, and until the end of the war, they got away with it.

In the case of abortion, the level of denial is similar and is accomplished by the dehumanization of the persons being killed. If you ask the question "Why are you killing those people?" one way to answer that question is "Those people are not really people." Those people are the moral equivalent of animals, or those people are people in the making but they haven't arrived at the point that they can be called "a person." Those are people who don't have the right to life or any other constitutional rights. Those people are uninvited guests. Those people are illicitly occupying someone else's body. Those people are in the way. Those people can, and in some cases should, be eliminated. In all these cases, we have a simple denial of the fact that the unborn human life is life worthy of protection, by the force not merely of public opinion but of law.

Second, we have an affirmation that even if the unborn are human beings, nevertheless, it is good for their mothers, their parents, and society to have the right and the choice, prior to birth, to be able to kill them. This is not a denial of the fact of what is going on, the fact that there is mass killing; this is an affirmation of the value of mass killing. Mass killing is a necessary thing. It is a justified thing. And it is even, in some ways, a good thing.

This is a debate that affects the deepest strains of our culture, and our world, with the highest of stakes. And yet it is a debate that has to be examined from all different sides and from the ground level. That is what I seek to do in this book. I frame the book around all the key arguments made by the pro-choice Left. I state them not as I would characterize them or as a pro-lifer would characterize them but in fact how the pro-choice Left frequently states their view. Then I examine the view in a balanced way and mount a critique of the view.

The truth is that we live in a society that prefers convenience, in which some women don't want to have their child. Men don't want to be responsible for being fathers. And other people don't want to deal with the societal burden. The child is in the way, and therefore it becomes targeted for assassination. This is the grim face of abortion. In this book, I face the reality of what is going on in this country, and I do not sugarcoat it. After examining and exposing it, countering rationalizations for abortion, I lay out how we as individuals can rise above this terrible evil and how society can abolish this plague from its midst. We did it in the case of slavery, and we are better for it. We can do it again.

A CLUSTER OF CELLS

"To be, or not to be, that is the question."[13]

—WILLIAM SHAKESPEARE, *Hamlet*

CHAPTER ONE

MYTH: Life begins when a baby is born. A fetus is just a cluster of cells. The fetus is only a potential human being, not a human being.

"Mommy's little cluster of cells"

—*Sign held by a little girl at a pro-life rally*

The critically acclaimed movie *Lady Bird* came out in 2017 and swept the country. The heroine of this coming-of-age story is a high school girl. In a key scene, she is listening to a presentation in her high school gym by someone who is pro-life and is showing pictures of body parts of aborted babies. Suddenly, our heroine interrupts the presentation by saying, "Just because something looks ugly doesn't mean it's morally wrong."

Then she adds, "If you took up-close pictures of my vagina while I am on my period, it would be disturbing, but it doesn't make it wrong." In her comments, she is likening the blood from her menstrual period to parts of an aborted baby, implying that the gruesome product of an abortion is nothing more than a cluster of cells. In making her comments, the heroine is addressing a woman who is sharing her story of how her own mother chose not to abort her and instead chose life. The heroine then says to the survivor, "If your mother had had the abortion, then we wouldn't have to sit through this stupid assembly."

Keep in mind that this rude girl is the heroine of this film, which received many accolades, including being nominated for multiple Oscars. The actress won a Golden Globe Award. The movie was named one of the ten best films of the year by *Time* magazine. This is a good example of how the cultural Left inserts this kind of messaging into everything—movies, songs, billboards, ads, TV shows, and sitcoms. The purpose is to normalize abortion, making the baby in the womb seem like nothing more than a cluster of cells.

But others far removed from the realm of popular culture assert this view as well. Supreme Court Justice John Paul Stevens, thirteen years after *Roe v. Wade*, wrote that "the nine-month fully gestated, fully sentient fetus on the eve of birth" is not a "human being."[14] His statement supports the Left's argument that having an abortion is no different than having your appendix or your tonsils removed. It's part of your body, but it's not a vital organ. If people have an appendix removed, they are fine. By their standards, the fetus is no different. It's a cluster of cells.

Before we can proceed, we must pose a basic question: What is pregnancy? What does it mean to be pregnant? When a woman takes a pregnancy test and the little stick comes up pink or is marked with a plus sign, what does this mean? Clearly something in her body has changed. We can all agree on that. She is getting morning sickness, her period stops, she's feeling tired, and her stomach is growing. Hmm. So let's take a look inside. Wow, the ultrasound is showing a tiny human in there! So, what is happening here?

Pregnancy is a state traditionally defined as being "with child." Does it mean to "be with a cluster of cells"? Let's see. *Merriam-Webster* defines the word "pregnant" as "containing a developing embryo, fetus, or unborn offspring within the body."[15] Ironically, the Guttmacher Institute, an affiliate of Planned Parenthood, has tried to muddy the waters as far as what the word "pregnant" means.[16] It titled an article "The Implications of Defining When a Woman Is Pregnant," and in it the author writes, "State definitions of pregnancy vary widely."[17] Strange! It seems obvious that pregnancy is biological, as we are literally seeing a physical change in the woman's body and the baby in the womb as well. Can the reality of pregnancy itself be determined by defining it differently? The Left is precisely trying to confuse us into thinking that pregnancy is not a biological state, is not medical, and does not involve a baby. The Left makes the "cluster of cells" argument to make the fetus seem like nothing.

What Change Has Occurred?

The abortion debate often revolves around the question—"When does life begin?" Let's take a step back from the abortion issue and think about regular life. All the time, people post pictures on social media, announcing "I'm pregnant" with captions like "Family of 3" with a photo of an ultrasound. Many young people post photos of their pregnancy and keep people updated as their baby develops. People hit the Like button and comment on the photos, usually writing "Congratulations!" or "I'm so excited for you!" People have gender-reveal parties and baby showers, inviting their family and friends. People feel the tummy of the woman, and when they feel a kick, they say, "She's going to be an active one!" or "What a big guy!"

Are these people simply delusional and living in their own world? Should they say, "You are with fetus" or "Nice cluster of cells"? When it comes to the abortion debate, we act like what's inside the woman's tummy is a big mystery; meanwhile, as we debate this issue and go back and forth, babies are born every day. They come into this world with their pudgy faces and scrunched-up eyes. And before you know it, they're crying, laughing, and walking, and they keep growing until they are the same size as the rest of us. So for us to act like the nature of the entity in the womb is entirely unknown to us is absurd.

What Is Life?

We must first establish that there is life in the womb when we are talking about a fetus. We are not talking about a rock. We are talking about something that has innate characteristics of life. But what is life? For decades, NASA has been looking for evidence of life on other planets, and it has located water on an exoplanet. It has made a breakthrough in finding both water vapor as well as temperatures that could sustain life. The planet, K2-18b, is eight times the size of Earth. One of the problems, however, is the planet is bombarded by radiation, far more radiation than Earth gets. While K2-18b may not sustain life, scientists are hopeful that there will be other exoplanets that can.[18]

The mission of the Seti Institute, which looks for signs of life on other planets, is "to explore, understand and explain the origin and nature of life in the universe and the evolution of intelligence."[19] When Seti finds the smallest signs of life on other planets, everyone from *National Geographic* to *Space* to the *New York Times* gets very excited. If anyone saw the signs of life that a fetus displays on another planet, we would go crazy because it's clearly life. If we saw these characteristics in something, we would know it's alive! Why would a microscopic speck of bacteria be considered life on Mars— and a heartbeat not be considered life on Earth?

We can easily open a biology textbook and learn the ingredients for life.[20] All living creatures are composed of cells. *Check.* They must be organized into different levels of complexity (cell, tissue, organ, organ system, organism, with higher organizations of populations and communities). *Check.* Living things have heredity. DNA is the molecule of heredity. *Check.* Living things have a metabolism. This means they take in energy for growth. They have homeostasis, which means they maintain a certain temperature. This is why we shiver when cold. They have the potential capacity to reproduce using DNA (sexual or asexual reproduction). They respond to the environment around them.

The fetus meets all of the signs of life. So we know there is life here and the fetus is in fact not equivalent to an appendix or a gallbladder. An appendix does not have heredity or a metabolism. It can never reproduce, no matter how old it is. It doesn't have a beating heart. You get the point.

What Is Human Life?

Now that we have established that the fetus has the characteristics of life, we must ask: What kind of life is it? When we talk about "right to life," we don't mean the right to life of a plant. We mean the right to life of a human. Human is a subcategory of life, a specific type of life we call human life. So, let's look at the different kinds of life there are. There are plants, mammals, fungi, protists, archaea, and bacteria. Within the category of "animal life" there are mammals, reptiles, birds, amphibians, and so on. We are mammals.

Okay, so is the fetus in the woman's body a reptile? I think not, since it's biologically impossible for two mammals to produce a reptile. Then is it a bird? Is it a plane? The point here is when we look into the nature of the fetus, we know it is life, and we know it is human life. Something that is inhuman does not become human as it gets older. Randy Alcorn, a *New York Times* best-selling author, puts it well: "Whatever is human, is human from the beginning."[21]

What Is a Cell?

Let's consider the Left's claim that "the fetus is a cluster of cells." What is a cell? In the book *The Way of the Cell*, we learn how complex the cell is. The cell is fully formed. It didn't evolve from something else because the cell is the most basic unit of life. This creation of new life is a kind of miracle. It's a natural miracle, but it's still a miracle that inspires marvel and wonder. "Wonder" is the appropriate word to apply to the cell. Scientists have worked hard to create cells and have come close—at least in appearance. Scientists at the University of California, San Diego (UCSD) have created "the most lifelike artificial cells yet."[22] Their latest pseudo-cells mimic the real thing and "look a little bit like natural cells, but they are made of completely artificial materials," says Henrike Niederholtmeyer, a synthetic biologist at UCSD.[23]

Encyclopedia Britannica defines a cell as "the basic membrane-bound unit that contains the fundamental molecules of life and of which all living things are composed. A single cell is often a complete organism in itself."[24] The U.S. National Library of Medicine says, "Cells are the basic building blocks of all living things. The human body is composed of trillions of cells. They provide structure for the body, take in nutrients from food, convert those nutrients into energy, and carry out specialized functions."[25] This shows that all of us are a cluster of cells. Literally. To say that the fetus is a cluster of cells is just as correct as saying you or I are a cluster of cells. It is not possible for life to exist without the clustering of cells.

The point of view that a fetus is a cluster of cells is the ultimate claim to justify abortion. The language dehumanizes the fetus and likens an abortion to removing your tonsils or your appendix, since not many view the cell in the complex fashion that scientists do. The real question we must ask is—Is the cluster of cells called the "fetus" identical to the cluster of cells called the woman? Let's turn to embryology to find out.

The Embryo

Since the advent of cell theory, developed by Matthias Schleiden and Theodor Schwann in 1839, we have known that the embryo develops from the single-celled zygote.[26] In 1859, the American Medical Association released a statement on the "independence of the zygote."[27] The zygote is not the father or the mother but its own unique entity. All of the cells in the woman, from her fingernail to her hair, are made up of her DNA, but the fetus's cells contain only half of her DNA and half of the father's DNA in order to create a unique result. There will never be another person with the same DNA as this person, even if the father and mother have another child or ten children. Even identical twins, who come from the same embryo, develop their own genetic reactions.[28] No being is identical to their mother or their father.

While the zygote is a cluster of cells, like you or me, it is more importantly an organism. Clusters of cells make up many things, including each of us as well as animals and plants. But an organism is an entity that is "an individual constituted to carry on the activities of life by means of organs separate in function but mutually dependent: a living being."[29] This view is held today by almost every embryologist. Even embryologists who are not remotely pro-life admit, as J. T. Eberl says, "As far as human 'life' per se, it is, for the most part, uncontroversial among the scientific and philosophical community that life begins at the moment when the genetic information contained in the sperm and the ovum combine to form a genetically unique cell." What Eberl finds controversial is "whether this genetically unique cell should be considered a human person."[30]

What Happens in the First Trimester

Let's turn to the first trimester and see how human the fetus is, by our own subjective adult human standards. "Moderate" pro-choice people sometimes take the position of life beginning at the second or third trimester, in an effort to put some limit on abortion while allowing it in the first trimester. For the same reason, some pro-lifers also make concessions here because by the second and third trimester it's a lot easier to convince someone of the fact that there is a human in there, one that's just like you and me.

The first trimester seems to be the most "invisible" aspect of pregnancy. Many of us hear about how developed a baby is in the second and third trimesters. From a clearly pregnant belly to a woman wearing maternity clothes to feeling the baby kick, there are so many ways in which the baby's life becomes concrete and visible to us. Except for morning sickness and other symptoms that may be clear to the woman and her doctor but not to a third-party observer, not much is going on in the first trimester. This then leads people to believe that fetal development begins much later. People don't think there's much of a "baby" in the first trimester, which then implies that first trimester abortions are not a big deal and are not the same as aborting a third-trimester infant.

This is actually what the medievals thought. They knew that having sex could lead to the conception of a child, but they didn't know if a child was conceived until they saw visible signs. They determined that life began at a point they informally called "quickening," which is the point when the woman can feel the baby kick. Naturally, they would then say, "Hey, there must be life in there!" Of course, they did not have anything near the medical technology we have today. Since there was little known about what went on internally in the female body, they decided that a baby was there when they could see the mother's pregnant belly and she could feel a kick in it.

If the woman had a large belly and there wasn't any sign of life inside, she could have just been a big lady. So feeling the baby kick was important to determining if it was there. But just because they determined life was there at the signs of kicking doesn't mean that philosophically they didn't value the sanctity of life. They just lacked medical knowledge—they didn't have ultrasound technology, embryology, and other scientific disciplines we have now.

Today, we have far more knowledge than they did, so we really can't claim ignorance. To focus only on life in the second and third trimesters would be to dismiss the significance of all of the development that occurs in the first trimester. Much to the naked eye's surprise, most of the major development of a human being actually occurs in the first trimester. Ever since the moment of conception, the baby's sex, hair color, eye color, and essentially all of its DNA are present. A unique set of DNA has been created and only develops from that point forward.[31]

According to Mayo Clinic, in the first trimester alone, the baby's toes, fingernails, bendable elbows, nose, head, hormones, and heartbeat develop.[32] Only eighteen days after conception, modern technology can detect the baby's heartbeat. We can see it beat after about twenty-two days. From this point onward, the heart never stops beating until the moment the person passes away and is declared dead. This heartbeat is a continuous one that goes on throughout life. In just the span of conception to birth, the baby's heart beats about fifty-four million times.[33] The blood its heart pumps is not blood from the mother but blood the baby has produced.[34] The heartbeat is the point at which we unequivocally know there is life there. And when there is no longer a continuing heartbeat, we know that life has ceased. This is the measure we use to determine life on Earth. To say that the baby is not a person when it has a heartbeat is counterintuitive to science and the system we use on Earth to "determine life."

About six weeks in, modern technology can detect the baby's brain waves.[35] The heartbeat and brain waves are both commonly referred to as "vital signs." Vital signs indicate whether someone is alive. If someone's heart stops beating and they are brain-dead, they are dead. However, the absence of only one of these vital signs means the person is alive. For example, if a person's heart is beating but their brain is not functioning, they are alive. Similarly, when a person's heart has stopped and needs to be revived while the brain is functioning, that person is considered alive. So for us to categorize a baby with a beating heart of its own as well as its own brain waves as "nothing more than a cluster of cells" or equivalent to an appendix would be factually incorrect.

By week six, the baby's fingers have formed on the hands.[36] Even though the woman usually doesn't feel it until later, the baby begins to spontaneously move around five to six weeks, into the pregnancy.[37] The baby can hiccup by seven weeks and the diaphragm muscle is completely formed, with intermittent breathing motions beginning.[38] About eight weeks into pregnancy, touching the baby will typically lead to squinting, jaw movement, grasping motions, and toe pointing.[39]

At about nine weeks in, the baby has developed a unique set of fingerprints. Doctors are able to distinguish the sex of the baby. This is typically when the parents find out the gender and you see gender announcements and gender reveals on social media. The baby is now producing its own reproductive cells. If it is a girl, she is already developing a uterus and ovaries. At about ten weeks in, the kidneys and gallbladder are functioning. By the twelfth week, the baby can cry.[40] All this development occurs in the first trimester alone.

By the end of the first trimester, the fetus now has every organ it will ever have, throughout its life, and development of these organs merely continues. Terms like "fetus" merely describe the stage of development the human is in. There are other stages of development like infant, toddler, teenager, or adult. We actually continue to develop for many years and the brain is not finished developing until we are about twenty-five years old. If a person is at a different developmental stage, then what we are discussing is an issue of form, not an issue of nature. The nature of the human is still human.

Let's think about the word "fetus." The Left loves to call a human in the womb a fetus instead of a human, even though the fetus is a human, because they want to dehumanize humans in the womb. The word "fetus" is Latin for "offspring." It doesn't mean "cluster of cells" or "potential human." "Offspring" has a meaning that we should think about. Clearly a fetus has not been born if it lives in the womb, but it already carries a title, "offspring," which we would apply to children that are born.

No one could possibly argue that human development begins once a baby is born. Clearly, development started before that, or else a fetus would come out of the womb without form—and certainly not with a beating heart. At one point every one of us was a fetus in the womb. We all were in that state and would not be able to be the people we are today if we had been killed at that stage of development. Regardless of where you stand on where life begins, we can all agree on what those lives become, which are small children or corpses.

CHAPTER TWO

MYTH: Even if it's technically a human life, the fetus doesn't feel anything or know what's happening anyway. As long as the fetus is dependent on the woman's body, we shouldn't consider it a separate life.

"Bliss was it in that dawn to be alive."[41]

—WILLIAM WORDSWORTH

Pro-choice advocates are quick to dismiss the moral anxiety over destroying unborn life on the grounds that the unborn don't really feel anything or know what is happening to them anyway. The fetus, like an animal, may have an instinct to survive, but it doesn't really know what death is. Our aversion to killing adult human beings is the anticipation of pain, loss of consciousness, and loss of independence. But pro-choice activists insist the unborn have none of this. They don't feel pain. They lack meaningful consciousness. They can't survive on their own outside the womb. In the course of an abortion, the only person who feels something or knows what's happening is the mother. Fetuses may be human, but pain, consciousness, and viability are important human characteristics to determine whether they indeed have the right to life.

Pain

The issue of fetal pain is often brought up by pro-choice advocates. They cite doctors who say, "A fetus can't feel pain!" and thereby conclude that if someone cannot feel pain, they are thereby not a person. But even if the fetus could not feel pain and if all data showing it does feel pain was completely ignored, this would not justify destroying its body and taking its life. Just because someone doesn't feel pain doesn't make it okay for you to do whatever you want with them, including killing them.

There are many who do not feel pain and who are clearly alive by any standard. Take someone who is paralyzed—are you half a person because half of your body doesn't feel pain? Does that mean that it is okay to burn that person's legs, since they can't feel pain in their legs, but to not do so to the part of them that can feel pain since that is the criterion in question? It is ridiculous to use "pain" as a criterion for determining if someone deserves to be harmed.

There are many who report feeling pain in a limb even when they have lost that limb. This is often referred to as a "phantom limb." The fact that over 80 percent of people with a phantom limb report feeling pain in that limb, when doctors are not exactly sure why, shows us that not all pain can be explained by doctors. Pain is somewhat subjective and applies to the person experiencing it. Pain is not something that another person can say, "Yes, you feel pain" or "No, you don't feel pain" because, ultimately, only you know when you feel pain. It is difficult to ask those in the womb how much pain they are in, but just as with a newborn infant or any person who cannot advocate for themselves, we can look at the signs they do express to see how much pain they are in. We can clearly judge when they are in pain based on what we do know.

Doctors used to think that the fetus could not feel pain until about twenty-four weeks. But now we have discovered that the fetus can feel pain at thirteen weeks.[42] How do we know this? The baby in the womb reacts to an invasive procedure with physical responses. When an abortion is attempted, the baby reacts with stress responses like increased cortisol showing that it is under duress. Whenever any of us are under duress, we do the same thing.[43]

It is puzzling to many in the medical field of neurology that the fetus can feel pain at thirteen weeks, since its neural pathways are not fully developed. Dr. Mark Rosen, who wrote an analysis of the fetal pain issue for the American Medical Association, is baffled by how the fetus can feel pain neurologically, since its pathways are not fully developed. He wrote that the cortex develops around the twenty-third week and continues developing after birth.[44] Dr. Nicholas Fisk, a fetal medicine specialist at Royal Brisbane and Women's Hospital in Australia, concurred regarding the development of the neural pathways, but he noticed that fetuses undergoing something invasive like a blood transfusion produced increased stress hormones and blood flow to the brain in those instances as well, but if given painkillers, these levels lowered.[45] If the fetus needs a painkiller before an abortion, what does this say about the pain we are causing it?

Dr. Kanwaljeet Anand, a professor of pediatrics, anesthesiology, and neurobiology at the University of Tennessee's Health Science

Center, studied the issue of fetal pain and found that not anesthetizing premature infants undergoing surgery caused the infants to produce stress responses from the brain as well and, outside of instances of abortion, resulted in an impeded recovery for the infant.[46]

In an article for *Behavioral and Brain Sciences*, Swedish neurologist Dr. Bjorn Merker discussed his observations of five children with hydranencephaly, a condition in which either most or all of the cortex of their brain was missing and instead replaced with fluid. He found that the children smiled, cried, and expressed pain. He wrote, "The tacit consensus concerning the cerebral cortex as the 'organ of consciousness'" may "be seriously in error."[47] Many adults continue to feel pain even after cortex tissue is removed. Overwhelming evidence shows us that the fetus does in fact feel pain, as early as thirteen weeks, even before the cortex develops.

Dr. Stuart Derbyshire, a prominent pro-choice physician from the United Kingdom, argues that since overwhelming evidence points to the fetus feeling pain at thirteen weeks, a form of anesthesia should be used on the infant before killing it in an abortion.[48] In a paper he cowrote with John C. Bockmann in the *Journal of Medical Ethics*, Derbyshire stated that "we are not currently aware of any procedures where invasive fetal intervention proceeds without anesthesia or analgesia, except for abortion."[49] While these studies continue to come out, leaders of pro-choice organizations continue to ignore them and assert that the fetus cannot feel pain until twenty-four weeks. Clare Murphy, of the British Pregnancy Advisory Service, the UK's largest abortion provider, refuses to accept these facts and instead repeats, "The most comprehensive review of this issue to date concluded a fetus cannot experience pain before 24 weeks."[50]

When we step outside the abortion debate, we see that it is clear that babies respond to outside stimuli and feel sensation at a mere fifteen weeks, gestation. For example, the popular book *What to Expect When You're Expecting*, read by millions of women every year, explains that at week fifteen the baby is sensitive to touch, stating "in fact, he or she will squirm if you poke your belly."[51] We also see at week fifteen that the baby is working on its "coordination, strength, and smarts to wiggle his or her fingers and toes and even suck a thumb," adding that while the mother can unlikely feel it yet, the baby is "kicking, flexing, and moving those arms and legs."[52]

We can actually see visible avoidance reactions from the baby during an abortion, even prior to thirteen weeks. The most common type of abortion method is where the fetus is sucked out of the womb through a suction tube. This can be done up to thirteen to fourteen weeks into pregnancy. I will explain the different types of abortion methods in more detail later on in the book, but this method is where a vacuum aspirator or another form of high-powered suction is inserted into the womb at ten to twenty times the force of a household vacuum cleaner in order to suck out the baby's limbs, brains, and heart. When the suction tube moves toward the baby in the womb, the baby literally tries to get away from the lethal object coming toward it—squirming and trapped with nowhere else to go. Even when a baby is very tiny, it does this. You may ask, does this really happen? How do we know it happens? And the answer is yes, it does happen, and we know this because we can see it on an ultrasound.

Abby Johnson, the director of a Planned Parenthood clinic in Bryan, Texas, saw this happen. She was a pro-choice advocate and one of Planned Parenthood's rising stars. Aside from her advocacy in speaking to women seeking abortions and administrative work in the clinic, she had never seen an abortion done in the operating room. One day she was asked to help out with an abortion. So, she went into the operating room and watched on an ultrasound as the abortionist performed the procedure. For the first time, she watched the suction tube make thrusting motions as it approached the baby. She watched as the baby tried to get away. Abby could not believe her eyes. She had always thought that a fetus at this stage was a cluster of cells. But she saw the baby move away in the womb, and saw that babies in the womb are literally capable of fighting for their lives, doing everything they can to survive.

Today, with the power of sonograms we don't have to take this on faith; we can see the baby do this in the womb. As depicted in the film *Unplanned*, Abby is horrified at what she sees, runs to a bathroom, and breaks down in tears. The film tells Abby's awe-inspiring conversion story. When the film shows the baby in the womb move away from the suction tube coming after it, you cannot help but shudder. It is heartbreaking and leaves one wondering how abortion doctors have calmly watched this scene happen for years. This is why many abortion clinics do not want women to see this happening in the ultrasound. The suction method of abortion is the most common way to abort a baby in the United States.

If a baby can express visible avoidance reactions to pain prior to thirteen weeks, is confirmed to feel pain at thirteen weeks by medical doctors, and is believed to feel pain at twenty-four weeks even by the far Left, then why are abortions still performed after twenty-four weeks? The pro-choice Left continues to justify abortions performed after this point, showing that fetal pain is not a factor that would stop them from aborting an infant.

Unbelievably, even some who acknowledge the fact that the

fetus does feel pain still think it's okay to abort this sentient living human being. Dr. Anand, for example, who says that pain is a real likelihood for the fetus, states that "the issue of fetal pain does not have much relevance for abortion."[53] He explains that technology could easily be used to prevent the fetus from feeling pain. The argument goes something like this: If we abort them in a quick way where they don't feel pain, it's okay. If it makes you feel better, you can use anesthesia on them so they don't feel pain while you abort them.

The fact that a doctor is saying that an infant can feel pain but we can abort it anyway shows us that fetal pain is not really the issue for the Left. Many don't care if the infant feels pain. Sadly, anesthesia is rarely administered on the infant being aborted, and not just in the first trimester but even in the second or third trimester on a late-term abortion, when the baby can kick and cry. The fact that someone has a shared humanity with us and has the ability to suffer means they are like us. So, if this does not justify their right to life, then what does? Just because you can pump someone with morphine doesn't mean you can kill them while you do it. Anthony McCarthy, a pro-life physician, states that "making death painless for the one killed does not, however, mean that taking life is thereby justified."[54]

Some on the Left argue that the fetus doesn't mind pain, since undergoing the passage through the birth canal involves pain as well. All I can say in response to this is that traveling through a birth canal is the opposite of being aborted. One procedure, giving birth, leads to life for the baby, while the other, the abortion, leads to its death. The baby positions itself on its head in order to travel through the birth canal, and this is a natural process, whereas the pain associated with abortion is completely unnatural.

It is traumatic for the baby to travel through the birth canal, and after traveling through the canal, the child comes into the world in an uncomfortable state, having left a warm and enclosed area. The baby's first howl is a good indicator of how uncomfortable it feels. This feeling of discomfort for the child in the birth process is not the same as injecting it with saline to die, suctioning it through a tube, and discarding it as waste. Abortion undoubtedly involves far more suffering for the baby.

Consciousness

Some argue that the baby is not a person because they don't believe it is conscious. They say, "Even if babies are human, no harm is done to them in the abortion process because they don't know about it."

In just the first few weeks in the womb, the fetus's neural tube gives rise to neurons and other cells of the central nervous system. At the same time, the central canal of the spinal cord is developing. The fetus is developing specific sections of the brain that will be used for the rest of its life.[55] This is acknowledged by medical doctors, associations, and even the *New York Times*. As early as the fifth to sixth week, the fetus's synapses are already developed enough to allow messaging to go to its brain, including messages to move.[56] In the seventh week, very early on in pregnancy, the baby's brain is producing brain cells at the rate of nearly one hundred per minute.[57] At this point, even the baby's kidneys are functioning to deal with its own waste management, namely, urine.[58] The baby performs coordinated actions like hiccupping, stretching, yawning, swallowing, and grasping. These tasks are fairly complex motor movements that involve a muscle connection to the brain. The fetus's brain develops at such a rapid pace that if a mother has an abortion even at ten weeks, the abortionist will feel a larger object, the baby's head and brain, and will have to crush it specifically with a metal device.

So, if the baby has a heartbeat and a brain by five to six weeks, performs motor skills, responds to stimuli, and emits the same stress responses as you and I do under duress, how can any argument be made to justify killing it? You would think the argument would end here because medical facts point to the fetus's humanity.

Let's look at consciousness, since the Left often questions the *level* of consciousness and exactly how complex it is. If human beings go into an unconscious state, can we kill them off? Many of us go through periods of not being conscious throughout our life. This happens anytime you have a surgery when you undergo anesthesia—say, when you get your wisdom teeth out, for example, or get a colonoscopy. What about athletes who have gotten a concussion from playing a game? We all lose a degree of consciousness every night when we fall asleep. But that doesn't warrant the killing of a sleeping person awaiting an alarm clock to go off. The baby in the womb is awaiting the alarm clock indicating it's time to come out of there. Is it right to kill them while they're waiting?

Some people liken the state of the fetus to that of a person in a coma, as if the fetus is a vegetable. This assumes that both the fetus and the person in the coma are unconscious. But it's important to remember that many babies in the womb have more brain activity than comatose people as well as more vital signs. Without outside interference to end the baby's life in the womb, this baby will keep growing and only become more conscious. As the infant in the womb keeps developing, their brain does as well, which is not always the case for the comatose person.

The comatose state of an adult raises the question of whether this person will be on life support forever. But the developmental stage of a human in the womb does not last forever. We know this. In fact, we know pretty accurately when it will be ready to exit the womb, which is a fixed period of time, nine months to be specific. This is a temporary stage not just for some infants but for all infants. In due time, the infant will be very present in this world and demanding constant attention.

When a spouse or the grown children choose not to keep an aged person on life support forever, they're assuming that the person would have made the same choice if they were in the position to do so. In this decision, the family members' decision is made for the person's welfare, not for the family's convenience. (Hospitals are warned against situations in which family members want to "pull the plug" on someone before it is time and often do not consider an ailing person making this decision to be mentally able to do so.) The choice here in the case of abortion is obviously completely different because any person coming into this world, with their entire life ahead of them, would not choose to be killed. Killing is clearly not in the best interest of the fetus.

It is also not the natural course of things, since in abortion the fetus is directly targeted, whether that be with an abortion pill that flushes it out of the mother's womb through a painful and bloody process, a suction that removes the fetus from the womb along with scraping out the rest of its body parts, or a needle injecting poison into the baby's heart. No one could fathom directly targeting and killing a comatose person in this brutal manner.

This is not to say that taking someone in a coma off life support is acceptable, but the point is that the position of the fetus and the position of a comatose person, so often compared, are actually radically different, and the comparison does not justify abortion.

In addition to consciousness, there is also cognition. How smart is this baby? Even if it's "conscious" how do we know it is cognitive? It is not able to make decisions and doesn't have moral reasoning skills as you or I do. Pro-abortion advocates argue that the fetus does not have a sense of life goals or purpose, if you will. However, this is another bad argument since this high level of cognition is not a standard that a three-week-old newborn, three-month-old infant, or three-year-old toddler would be able to meet. I am not sure many other twenty-somethings have their life purpose figured out either, let alone a complex direction for their life. This is clearly the case for old people after a certain age, as priorities shift from life goals to memories and enjoying one's present time on Earth.

Regarding the baby in the womb, it actually does have a sense of relationships as well as the ability to learn. Why do you think women are encouraged to speak to their baby in the womb? Because it can hear you. Experts in fetal development confirm that speaking to the baby in utero helps with its language development, as babies can even begin to remember words in the third trimester.[59] Similarly, when a baby is born, it recognizes the sound of its mother's voice, even when its eyes remain closed. The baby often recognizes the voice of the father as well.

It is remarkable that doctors are even able to perform brain surgery on infants born prematurely, showing us that their brain development is quite complex and similar to ours. Dr. Ben Carson has performed brain surgery on twenty-five-week-old babies. In an appearance on *The View* in 2015, Carson said, "I've spent my entire career trying to preserve life and give people quality of life, even operating on babies in the womb, operating all night long sometimes on premature babies." Carson continued, "And I get to meet those people when they're adults, and productive adults. There is no way you're going to convince me that they're not important."[60] Ben Carson was the first neurosurgeon to separate conjoined twins, which are twins who become physically attached to each other during their development in the womb.

Whenever I hear people argue that the fetus is not "human enough" because it doesn't have complex moral reasoning skills and so on, I think of a newborn infant. Infants certainly don't have deep thoughts or moral reasoning skills. They don't have dreams for their future, and they aren't making plans. A newborn infant is far more similar in its level of consciousness to a fetus in the womb than to a fully grown adult. But if I saw you kill an infant, I would be horrified.

Even if we think of our pets that have humanlike qualities, we wouldn't want to torture them. If I saw you walk up to your dog and start kicking it, I would shudder. I think we all would. Why? Because some aspect of them feels something, and some aspect of them knows something is harming them, and that's bad. The child in the womb and the child once born are not very different from one another. And the fetus clearly is more morally worthy of humane treatment than any animal, by virtue of being human, but if we are willing to protect our pets from being tortured, then why not babies? Animals and humans should not be compared, but I draw this comparison because so many of us would jump out of our seats if we saw someone torturing our pet. Infanticide is wrong, and brutally torturing your pet is wrong, so why is torturing a baby in the womb morally acceptable?

Viability

Pro-choice activists often make the argument that says, "As long as the fetus is dependent on the woman's body, we shouldn't consider it a separate life. Women should be able to get abortions up to the point of viability. Once the baby is viable it is a separate entity with separate claims." Some argue that the baby is not a person because it is dependent on the mother. This then leads some to take the view that the baby only becomes a person when it is viable, meaning it can live on its own outside the mother. Until then, it is an extension of the woman's body.

While this is a popular opinion embraced in the Supreme Court's *Roe v. Wade* decision, it does not make sense. If a baby is only considered a "living person" once it is "independent," then we must admit that most living people are not actually living people because they are still dependent on others. A newborn baby is dependent on its mother every few hours for milk and nutrients and needs constant care. If you leave an infant on the floor and do not tend to it, it will die. To say it is "independent" would be incorrect. A toddler is hardly independent. As children get older, they become more independent and are able to feed themselves, but parents usually provide food and shelter for their children until they take off on their own for work or college.

Also consider that many adults are not physically independent in that they rely on some outside aid in order to survive. Think of all of the people who have pacemakers. Not to mention, there are elderly people in assisted living homes on feeding tubes, literally getting their nourishment from an outside source. A person on life support who cannot survive without the machine and the doctor is certainly not "viable." So to say that to be a "person" you must be "viable" really doesn't work, as millions of Americans would not meet that standard.

We also must acknowledge medical facts, which is to say that the relationship between mother and fetus is not a one-way street. The baby is not sucking the life out of the mother while growing inside her. The baby has developed its own blood and is pumping it with its own heart. In the womb, the fetus receives blood proteins from the mother that protect it from diseases for the rest of its life, but this relationship is symbiotic. When the mother suffers organ damage or a heart attack, for example, the fetus sends stem cells through the placenta to repair her damaged organ. This is called fetomaternal microchimerism. This is not a voluntary action taken by the fetus but happens on its own, as when nutrients from the mother are involuntarily sent to the fetus. Identical twins can also exchange microchimeric cells through the placenta in order to strengthen one another.[61]

These cells that are exchanged between fetus and mother often stay in the mother past giving birth, aiding her with future ailments. An article in *Scientific American* says, "Evidence is building that those fetal cells aren't just lounging around in Mom; in fact, they might be active participants in a mother's health." Recent studies suggest that these fetal cells that reside in Mom can even help prevent her from developing autoimmune disorders, such as rheumatoid arthritis, and are likely caused "by the mother's immune response to the child's cells."[62] The article says, "Fetal cells also appear to migrate to injury sites and have been found in patients with thyroid and liver damage, where they had morphed into organ cells, which suggests that they are on a repair mission."[63] This is likely because many of these microchimeric cells are stem cells, which can reproduce indefinitely and transform into other types of tissue. Fetal stem cells in a mother's body help her heal.

In *Circulation Research*, a journal of the American Heart Association, an article subtitled "Baby Gives Back" reported on a study of the effect of microchimeric cells, which found that fetal cells are typically found at the site of injury in a mother and "fetal cell microchimerism has been repeatedly demonstrated in rodent models, primates, and humans." This is a major biological difference between women and men. It states, "On a more human level, it is fascinating to realize that after the mother spends nine months providing nutrients and an environment for optimal growth and development of the baby, the baby gives back cells with regenerative potential to the mother."[64]

Let's get back to viability. To say that the point of viability is "when life begins" is arbitrary because the point of viability continues to get earlier and earlier as medical technology advances. There is no specific point in time. If you had asked someone a hundred years ago what the point of viability is, they wouldn't know or would probably tell you whenever the baby is born. Now, babies can be born at twenty-one weeks with advanced premature natal care. Twins are often born early, triplets earlier, and quadruplets even earlier all of which is very typical. When discussing viability, we also must realize that there is induced labor, where the woman gives birth early, making viability even more arbitrary because sometimes doctors can choose when the baby is delivered.

The point of viability for the fetus also depends on the advancement of medical technology and the medical capabilities of the particular hospital visited by the mother, making it even more arbitrary.[65] Advancing medical technology in this arena is not something *Roe v. Wade* took into account. There is a provision in *Roe v. Wade* that deals with viability and warns that abortion is more problematic once a baby is viable. This shows that what they were ruling on in 1973 is completely different from now. Even Supreme Court Justice Ruth Bader Ginsburg considers the "viability" argument to be shaky. She says, "Overall, the Court's *Roe* position is weakened, I believe, by the opinion's concentration on a medically approved autonomy idea."[66]

I would also like to point out that even if you think the fetus is not a life until it is viable, this is no longer the position of the Democrats, as it was in the wake of *Roe v. Wade* in the seventies. The Democratic Party platform finds abortion without a medical reason acceptable at nine months, up to the point of birth. The Democratic Party Platform states: "We will continue to oppose—and seek to overturn—federal and state laws and policies that impede a woman's access to abortion."[67] Only allowing abortion to the point of "viability" is not a position that Democrats hold today, and if you are a Democrat in elected office who thinks this, you will likely be shunned and publicly shamed by your own party because you are invalidating abortions that would take place after the point of viability, and this is something the Democrats will not concede on. Hillary Clinton, Elizabeth Warren, Bernie Sanders, Pete Buttigieg, and all of the most prominent and powerful Democrat politicians are on board with this extreme position.

Perhaps you think viability is no longer a good argument because of how arbitrary it is. Some believe that a baby is only a baby once it's born, but this then raises the question—Should stillborn babies be considered "babies" at all? They were alive in the womb but upon exiting the womb are not alive. Under the "person at birth" logic, these babies would not be babies at all. Doctors refer to stillborn babies as babies who have died. They do not refer to them as a cluster of cells or a nonperson. The common practice is that once a stillborn baby is born, the baby is cleansed, measured, and given a name. The mother is given the opportunity to hold the baby.[68] The fact that the baby was once alive in the womb but never after birth does not mean that it was never a human. And this is not my opinion. This is how the medical community views it and treats it; I am just relaying this information.[69]

Maybe you think that point of birth is an unambiguous point at which we can determine "life begins," but in fact there is ambiguity about even this. Is the baby a life when part of the baby is outside the mother's body? When the entire baby is outside? Or when the placenta is removed from the womb?[70] If you genuinely argue that "point of birth" is the moment when life begins, you must acknowledge that there are multiple "points" in birth. You may find this line of questioning silly, but that is only because the baby is so obviously human at any of these points. Do moments before or after birth make a difference to this shriveled-up, pudgy child? We must acknowledge that the only real difference between any of these situations is a matter of the baby's location.

Peter Singer, philosopher and bioethics professor at Princeton University, concedes that this is a valid point. He realizes that there isn't much of a difference between a preborn infant and a one-day-old infant or even a fifteen-day-old infant. The only real difference is its location, since developmentally they are virtually the same. He thinks that all preborn infants, as well as newborn infants up to twenty-eight days old, should be subject to termination or, rather, infanticide. Singer writes in response to the question "Should the baby live?" that "a period of twenty-eight days after birth might be allowed before an infant is accepted as having the same right to life as others."[71]

Some argue that the fetus gets more and more rights as it develops. So if it is six months along, it will not have as many rights as when it is eight months along. However, as we know, usually the question is one of life or death for the fetus, so there isn't a situation where a continuum of value placed on its life would matter.

Someone may then pick a point that doesn't depend on pain, consciousness, or viability. They may pick a point along development, like the heartbeat, lung function, or brain function, as the moment "when life begins." But this doesn't work either. To quote Ben Shapiro from his appearance on *EWTN Pro Life Weekly*, "Is it with a heartbeat? Because there are plenty of people living on a pacemaker. Is it with lung function? Because there are plenty of people living on iron lungs. Is it with brain function? Because you're asleep sometimes, and when you're a newborn baby your own brain function isn't particularly high."[72] We see that if we pick any of these arbitrary points in development as "the key," many of us could not meet the standard. In any case, life doesn't begin at a point when you say arbitrarily to the fetus, "Okay it begins!"

We have to begin at the beginning. From the moment a unique life is created with its own DNA, you have a unique organism. It is implanted and continues to develop rapidly. We find ourselves between a rock and a hard place if we want to pick a later point for "life beginning." If you are going to pick a point where "life begins" along its development, you could technically pick anywhere until age twenty-five, since that's when we are fully developed.

In sum, not having cognition and awareness of the world

around us is not a legitimate justification for killing. A person's level of pain tolerance does not permit us to do anything we want to them. Neither does the person's level of consciousness. Here are some facts: If you kill a preborn sea turtle, you get a $100,000 fine and one year in prison. If you kill a preborn bald eagle, you get a $250,000 fine and two years in prison. Yet a human in the womb can be killed on demand.

Let's pause and think about that. Is a preborn sea turtle more conscious than the fetus? Does a preborn bald eagle feel more pain than the fetus? No. Clearly our society puts greater value on preborn sea turtles and bald eagles than on preborn humans. This also shows us that all arguments made about pain, consciousness, or viability regarding the fetus are simply fronts to justify abortion. Very few pro-choice people really care if the fetus feels pain, is conscious, or is viable because if they did, they would be protesting these other ridiculous laws about sea turtles and bald eagles. Yet they advocate for those laws and, at the same time, advocate to strike down any law preventing the killing of a fetus that feels pain, is conscious, and is viable.

Many believe that the fetus was made "in God's likeness" and this is true, but it is also made in our likeness. Specifically, the likeness of its parents. More broadly, the fetus is also made in the likeness of every human, as we have all been through the same developmental stages. Is that not enough to show us its humanity? Are we so cold as to dehumanize them even when we've all been in their position in our early lives, in order to be the people we are today?

CHAPTER THREE

MYTH: There is a difference between a human being and a person. Even if the fetus is human, it is not a person with rights.

> "We hold these truths to be self-evident, that all men are created equal, that they are endowed by their Creator with certain unalienable rights, that among these are life, liberty, and the pursuit of happiness."
>
> —*Declaration of Independence*, 1776

We have established definitively that the unborn "cluster of cells" is human. This can hardly be doubted. And so the pro-choice argument begins to shift from the "cluster of cells" argument to the "they may be a human, but they're not a person" argument. This argument concedes the humanity of the unborn but denies their personhood, thus laying the groundwork to argue that the Founders never intended for rights to apply to the unborn. When we read the Constitution, the Constitution speaks of persons. The Fifth Amendment, for example, talks about the due process rights of persons. The Fourteenth Amendment speaks of equal protection of the laws, which applies to persons. This creates an opening for abortion advocates to say that human beings are different from persons. While being human is a given, "personhood" is a special status. So, our rights—our right to life, our right to liberty—accrue not to human beings per se but only to persons as understood in the eyes of the law.

In this view, our rights are conferred by the law, which is to say, by the Constitution. And so the law, and indeed society, can determine who has rights and who doesn't. Rights become something that is granted not by a higher power but by the state. And if the state decides that some people should have rights, then they do; and if the state decides others should not have rights, then they don't. Pro-choice advocates typically see personhood as something that can be debated, as something that is arbitrary.

Some say personhood is achieved at the moment of birth, which is worth thinking about: a human baby spends nine months in the womb as "a cluster of cells" and then *poof*, he or she is a person at the moment of birth. Others say personhood is achieved when the baby becomes "viable"—a point that is always shifting around on the gestational timetable. Still others say it is a continuum, where the fetus gets more rights as it develops. Under this thinking, a baby who is one month old has less value than a baby who is eight months old because the eight-month-old has been around longer. And so rights, in a sense, drop in wherever it suits the advocate. There is a time when this human becomes a person and attains rights. Before that, they have no rights. Such mental gymnastics are mind-numbing.

Hillary Clinton has said she believes that rights of personhood begin only at birth. Her words when she was running for president in 2016: "The unborn person doesn't have constitutional rights."[73] Those who are pro-life found this morally wrong and emotionally cold. Even those who are pro-choice and in Hillary's camp criticized her because she made the unforgivable mistake of referring to the unborn as "a person." The Left knows that as soon you refer to someone as a person, even by accident because it just slipped out, it becomes problematic to argue that the baby can be lawfully killed at whim. This pro-choice argument denies that there is such a thing as intrinsic or inalienable rights. There are only the rights that are conferred by the state. *Roe v. Wade*, in a sense, proclaims the non-personhood of the fetus prior to viability.

So let's consider the question—What is the difference between human beings and persons? If we really think about these two terms, we realize that they are indistinguishable. In other words, there is no difference between a human being and a person. When it comes to your human rights or your basic or natural rights, all human beings are persons, and all persons are human beings.

As soon as we differentiate between "humans" and "persons," we have set the stage for man's most perverse horrors. This is the justification the Nazis used, claiming that Jews are humans but not persons. This is the justification used for slavery, claiming that blacks are humans but not persons. By saying someone is a human but not a person, you are saying you have the right to do with them as you wish—torturing them, killing them, using their skin for lampshades. And indeed, this is exactly what the Left argues can be done to the human in the womb, airily saying that "it may be a human, but it doesn't embody personhood."

Let's look at the idea of whether personhood is a continuum. Certainly, an eight-month-old baby has a higher sense of awareness and cognition than a one-month-old baby, but does that make the eight-month-old infant more valuable than a one-month-old infant? No, of course not. A twelve-year-old is no more valuable as a person than a nine-year-old. If you have two children—one of them twelve, the other nine—you're not going to say that the twelve-year-old has a greater right to life than the nine-year-old. That would be absurd.

And, of course, this applies at the other end of life as well. For example, to say that the penalty for killing a seventy-five-year-old should be less than the penalty for killing a fifty-year-old would make no sense. In both cases, it's murder and the penalty is the same because the crimes are the same. The law doesn't put a different value on the life you took based on age or gender, but what the law does take into account is whether the murder was premeditated or accidental, and so on. The crime is the taking of innocent human life. Human lives have equal value when you are talking about murder.

To be sure, some types of rights depend on age and maturity, which is to say that there is legal acknowledgment of the continuum idea. Consider, for example, the matter of driving. A ten-year-old does not have the authority to drive, but a sixteen-year-old who has passed the driving test can. A ten-year-old cannot vote, but an eighteen-year-old can. It isn't hard to understand that as we reach certain points of maturity, we are eligible to partake in certain activities that we were not eligible to do at an earlier stage of our lives.

What we're talking about here is an important distinction between natural rights on the one hand and civil rights on the other. Civil rights, of course, are rights conferred by the state. But here I want to focus on natural rights, which are different from civil rights. Natural rights are rights that we have by virtue of being human; just by virtue of being a person. These are rights that we have, you may say, prior to being part of a civil community. These are rights that we have, as the early modern philosophers used to say, in the state of nature. That's why the Declaration of Independence calls these rights—the right to life, the right to liberty, and the right to the pursuit of happiness—inalienable. They're inalienable in the sense that we can't sell them or barter them away, even if we wanted to. America's very foundation is rooted in these inalienable rights.

Let's turn to the Founders for a moment to see where they believed our rights come from. Interestingly, Thomas Jefferson, who was a man of the Enlightenment and one of the least religious of the Founders, says that our rights come from our Creator. Our rights, in other words, come from our being God's anointed creation and superior to all other living creatures. It seems that one could dismiss this argument today as being somewhat antiquated, but it's pretty hard to think of where else such profound rights come from. In my view, what distinguishes human beings from other animals is that we are moral creatures.

We are creatures that have a moral status different from other animals. Natural rights, for the Founders, are the rights that you are born with. Natural rights and human rights are also a universal aspiration that transcend the whims of governments constructed by men. Consider, for example, the list of human rights listed in the United Nations' Universal Declaration of Human Rights. One of these is the right, for example, not to be tortured. Another is the right, as a civilian, not to be targeted in war. Governments may or may not respect or recognize these rights, but the point of the UN declaration is that these rights exist, and to violate them is to commit a high crime against human rights.

Thomas Hobbes, the English philosopher who conceived of a virtually all-powerful state, says that we turn over our rights to the state when we enter a social compact. But, he argues, we only owe allegiance to the state when it protects our life and safety. And if the state doesn't give us the right to life, then we have every cause to rebel and resist. In other words, we confer some of our rights to the state in exchange for protection of life, but when the protection is withheld or denied, then the deal is off. The right to life is the fundamental right. It is the right that ultimately makes all other rights possible. Without it, we have nothing. It is the most natural of natural rights, the most human of human rights.

These reasons are why we speak of the Right-to-Life movement. It is a movement that is fighting for the most basic right of all—life.

In the smoke-and-mirrors debate over whether a baby in the womb is a person or a human, the only truly important issue is obscured. What matters is that a baby—surely a human and surely a person—can be deprived under our laws of his or her right to life. It is a moral abomination before God and all civilized men and women.

Trying to distinguish a human from a person is a recipe for

tyranny, enslavement, and totalitarianism. We are human beings, and we are also persons. The unborn are human beings and also persons. Their worth, like our worth, does not come from society or the law or the state. They are God's littlest creatures and deserve the full protection of our nation.

CHAPTER FOUR

MYTH: Abortion is a simple and safe procedure, no different from any other medical procedure. Abortion is health care.

> "I will not give a lethal drug to anyone if I am asked, nor will I advise such a plan; and similarly, I will not give a woman a pessary to cause an abortion."
>
> —*Hippocratic Oath*[74]

Bernie Sanders tweeted on the day of the March for Life in 2020: "Abortion is health care."[75] Pennsylvania attorney general Josh Shapiro tweeted the same thing saying, "Abortion is healthcare."[76] Elizabeth Warren tweeted, also on the day of the March for Life, "Abortion is a healthcare right." We are bombarded with this messaging. It goes along with the familiar comment that "abortion is a simple and safe procedure." Planned Parenthood's official position: "Both in-clinic and medication abortions are very safe. In fact, abortion is one of the safest medical procedures out there."[77]

The National Abortion Federation (NAF) echoes this when it asserts, "Surgical abortion is one of the safest types of medical procedures."[78] After all, it implies, if it's just a cluster of cells and nothing more than a polyp, how difficult could removing it be? The Left likens abortion in the first trimester to abortion in the second trimester to abortion in the third trimester, since all are considered "health care." They find that aborting a baby at three months is no different from aborting it at eight months. The Center for American Progress has explained, "Late-term abortion is not a medical term It's a word made up by anti-choice opponents."[79]

What the Left is trying to do is make abortion at any month seem like "no big deal." It's just another procedure that doctors and medical professionals perform every day. This portrayal of abortion has plausibility in the medical community. I interviewed a gynecologist who is pro-life, and he admits that while he was in residency he performed abortions. It was presented to him as just another procedure. It was taught to him along with an array of other techniques in order to become a doctor. Abortion was presented to him as "health care," and it wasn't until later that he came to realize the reality of the procedure he was performing.

Democrats Oppose Women's Health Regulations

One would think that Democrats who call abortion health care and "a simple and safe procedure" would be looking out for women's health. But no, Democrats oppose health regulations when it comes to anything related to abortion. They oppose laws that make sure that the abortion facility is located near a hospital emergency room in case something unexpected occurs. If emergency care is not available, the woman could die. The Left also opposes regulations requiring that hallways in abortion clinics be wide enough to fit a stretcher in case it's needed in an emergency.[80]

Not being able to fit a stretcher into an abortion operating room is a serious hazard to a woman's health should she need to be transported to an emergency room. The infamous abortionist Kermit Gosnell performed countless abortions and was convicted for murder, since he also murdered babies outside the womb. He also harmed many women in the process. The grand jury report on his despicable operation states: "Ambulances were summoned to pick up the waiting patients, but...emergency personnel...discovered they could not maneuver stretchers through the building's narrow hallways to reach the patients....Gosnell's clinic, with its narrow, twisted passageways, could not accommodate a stretcher at all."[81]

Planned Parenthood is fighting hard against these health regulations. "At no point does the width of doorways have any bearing on the medical treatment that's being administered," says Planned Parenthood of Indiana executive director Betty Cockrum.[82] Planned Parenthood also states on their website that "there is no medical basis for [such] laws" as "a mandate that all abortion providers comply with onerous and medically unnecessary building requirements for ambulatory surgical centers (ASCs), and an unfair, also medically unnecessary requirement that doctors who provide abortions obtain hospital admitting privileges at a nearby hospital."[83]

This is precisely the issue that the Supreme Court examined this year. A Louisiana law stated that abortion clinics must be within thirty miles of a hospital and have admitting privileges there in case a woman having a surgical abortion procedure should need to be rushed to the emergency room. Abortion clinics themselves often don't have the medical equipment that full-fledged hospitals do, which is why access to emergency room care is needed should a life-threatening emergency arise. In a horrific 5–4 decision, the Supreme Court struck down this law, making it a win for pro-abortion advocates and loss for advocates of women's health.[84] This decision, and the Democrats' support of it, will go down in history as one of the most disgraceful decisions disregarding the health of women.

Is the Abortion Procedure That Simple or Safe?

In this chapter we are going to learn about how a baby is aborted. How does it actually happen? What methods and tools are used, and what happens to the grisly remains of the dismembered baby? You may be medically knowledgeable yourself and familiar with this information, but it's important to present this because many of the girls and women that go in for an abortion are not routinely informed about what is happening to them.

Normally, when you go in for a medical procedure, you get a detailed account of what is going to happen to you. But at abortion clinics like Planned Parenthood, the staff is reticent about the procedure because they, too, realize that the more detail they offer about the procedure, the less likely the woman is to go through with it. Their goal is to make it seem routine.

When a woman is seeking an abortion, she should know the several ways babies are aborted depending on their size. The four methods include:

1. Abortion pills
2. Suction D&C (dilatation and curettage); also known as suction curettage or vacuum aspiration

3. Dilation and evacuation (D&E)

4. Induction

You may hear the terms "medical" and "surgical" abortions. The term "medical abortion" applies only to the abortion pill because there is no surgery involved. All other abortions are "surgical" in that they require an operation conducted by an abortion doctor. The abortion pill can be taken up to ten weeks after the woman's last menstrual period. The suction method can be used up to sixteen weeks since a woman's last period. The D&E method is used after sixteen weeks.[85] The induction method is used after twenty-five weeks. These are all legal procedures that go on every day in America.

The Abortion Pill

The abortion pill method accounts for about 27 percent of abortions performed in America, according to the Centers for Disease Control and Prevention (CDC).[86] The abortion pill may seem the simplest and safest because you take it in the privacy of your own home and don't have to go under the knife. Planned Parenthood describes it on its website as "more natural" and "less invasive." Under the section "How Does the Abortion Pill Work?" it describes it as "kind of like having a really heavy, crampy period."[87] In other words, this should be nothing too intense, you'll be good. But what does the abortion pill actually do? Let's turn to science and medical facts.

Abortion pills consist of two things: mifepristone (RU486) and misoprostol. Mifepristone was first licensed in France and China in 1988.[88] By 1991 it was allowed in most European countries and was approved in the United States in 2000.[89] Mifepristone is taken first, in the presence of a medical professional and actually blocks the woman's progesterone, which stops the baby's development. At the same time, the uterus contracts and the cervix softens to allow expulsion."[90] The woman may feel nauseous and begin to experience bleeding.

Then, at home, up to forty-eight hours later, she takes the misoprostol. This causes severe cramping and bleeding to empty the uterus, expelling the fetus from the body. This is the part when it becomes extremely painful for the woman. She witnesses the abortion of her own baby, usually over the course of many hours as she bleeds out blood clots consisting of various parts of her baby. Planned Parenthood's website states that "it's normal to see large blood clots (up to the size of a lemon) or clumps of tissue when this is happening.... The cramping and bleeding can last for several hours.... The cramping and bleeding slow down after the pregnancy tissue comes out."[91]

In additional advice, the pro-abortion organization NAF explains that though the fetus is small and covered in blood, the woman may see a recognizable body including hands, fingers, and toes.[92] Bleeding and spotting can last for several weeks after the at-home abortion takes place.

Here's how one woman described her experience with the abortion pill to *Marie Claire* magazine:

[I expected] some cramping and bleeding, similar to or greater than a normal, heavy period. This sounded far more appealing than surgical abortion. A few pills, a couple of cramps, and it would all be over. We could move on with our lives.... Nothing—not the drug literature, the clinic doctor, not even my own gyno—had prepared me for the searing, gripping, squeezing pain that ripped through my belly 30 minutes later. I couldn't even form words when Stewart [her boyfriend] called to check on me. It was all I could do to gasp, 'Come home! Now!' For 90 minutes, I was disoriented, nauseated, and, between crushing waves of contractions, that I imagine were close to what labor feels like, racing from the bed to the bathroom with diarrhea....The next night, I started bleeding. I bled for 14 days.[93]

Another woman described her experience to *Cosmopolitan* magazine, saying, "Emotionally I was a wreck. I cried through the entire ordeal. I was so sad even though I knew it was the right thing to do right now....It's one of the most overwhelming experiences of my life."[94]

Another woman said, "I didn't expect the grief. It overwhelmed me....Every woman I have spoken to who had an abortion, regardless of their situation at the time, spoke of grief....It feels like you aren't allowed to grieve if it was your choice to do this."[95]

So many women feel like they can't talk about their grief, an emotion the pro-choice Left hates. This Leftist narrative that a fetus isn't a person leads women to suppress the very real pain that so many experience. Women who get abortions, who are not political activists, would not experience this grief and pain if they did not see what was happening to their body and what was coming out of them when they had the abortion. Pregnant women know what is inside them. It is maternal instinct. It's physically and emotionally painful to expel a dead fetus. This type of abortion, even the least invasive and supposedly most natural option, can leave emotional scars that last for many years.

We must also ask: Is the abortion pill safe? According to the FDA, heavy bleeding (heavier than a menstrual period) following the procedure is expected and about 8 percent of women experience it for thirty days thereafter.[96] In fact, if you don't experience bleeding, it is likely that the procedure has failed. Between 2.9–4.6 percent of women who take abortion pills at home end up in an emergency room as a result, according to the FDA.[97] About 3 percent of the time, women will need to have a surgical procedure to follow, in the event that the fetus is not fully aborted at home. If the fetus is not fully aborted and the woman does not have a follow-up surgical procedure, infection is likely to follow and is very dangerous. Other possible side effects include an ectopic pregnancy, and 12 percent of the time taking the pills does not produce an abortion and can lead to birth defects instead.[98] We will consider the cases where there are birth defects in another chapter, but now let's look at abortion by suction, the second type of abortion procedure.

Abortion by Suction

Abortion by suction is the most common way to abort a fetus. This is also called suction curettage or suction D&C (which stands for dilation and curettage). Suction curettage was first used in Russia in 1927, and the technique was perfected in China.[99] Abortion rates in Russia and China are some of the highest in the world to this day. This type of abortion is a surgical procedure and can only be performed on a woman in the first trimester. When undergoing this procedure, the woman needs to be anesthetized.

After anesthesia is administered, a speculum is placed inside the vagina, and the blades are widened to allow the doctor to view the cervix, which is the entrance to the uterus. During a normal pregnancy, the cervix is closed to protect the baby in the womb. But in order to perform a surgical abortion of any kind, the cervix must be opened so that the tools used for the abortion can get inside the opening and suck the baby out. If the cervix is forcibly dilated (opened), the woman can experience side effects like lacerations and perforations. The most common side effect is that future pregnancies are at risk due to trauma to the cervix. When you forcibly open the cervix during a surgical abortion and the cervix is intended to stay shut, you risk damaging the cervix, which is why the woman is at a higher risk of miscarriage in the future. When the cervix opens before it is supposed to, a miscarriage takes place.

Once the cervix is dilated, a cannula (tube) is inserted through the cervix and into the womb. The size of the tube used varies depending on how many weeks gestation the baby is in the womb. If a baby is at nine weeks gestation, typically a 9-inch catheter is used.[100] Some abortionists also have personal preference in catheter size. Some doctors choose to use a larger one for "ease and speed of uterine evacuation" and "more intact tissue," which aids the inspection process of the baby's body parts postabortion.[101] Others prefer to use a smaller catheter because it is less likely to harm the woman.

The tube is attached to a vacuum aspirator that operates at a suction force about ten to twenty times more powerful than a vacuum cleaner. The womb is intended to be a safe place for the baby, and yet it becomes a house of horrors with the abortionist's intrusion. There are two types of aspirators—a manual vacuum aspirator and an electric aspirator.[102] Even though the baby has a beating heart, a brain, head, fingers, and toes, its body parts are still very soft because its bones are still forming. This allows the suction to be able to pull the baby's organs through its tube. The suction pulls the baby apart, sucking out the parts, followed by the placenta. When doing a suction procedure, and watching the process via an ultrasound, you can often see the baby try to get away from the suction. When the suction comes after it, it moves in the womb, but with nowhere else to go because it is trapped.

However, one of the risks of suction method is incomplete abortion, meaning that parts of the baby or placenta are left behind, which can lead to complications like infection and abnormal bleeding. The tube is rotated and moved throughout the womb in order to get as many fetal parts as possible. Afterward, the abortionist uses a curette, a long-handled curved blade, to scrape the lining of the uterus to ensure that all parts have been removed. Once the baby parts have been suctioned, they are kept in a container that is carefully inspected to identify body parts. This body part identification process is standard procedure to make sure that all of the baby was torn apart and removed from the woman. There are some less common side effects to this procedure like injury to neighboring organs including the intestine, bladder, and blood vessels. Other risks include hemorrhage, infection, and, in rare cases, death. In addition, the psychological and emotional impact can be horrendous.

Abortion by Dilation and Evacuation

Abortion by D&E is a surgical abortion procedure done on pregnancies in the second trimester and sometimes in the third trimester. This procedure involves extreme dilation of the cervix because of the baby's larger size. With the woman under anesthesia, the cervix is dilated using metal dilators and a speculum. The abortionist then inserts a suction catheter to empty out any fluid. At this stage, the baby is a well-formed and sturdy entity with bones and a fairly hard cranium, so the suction will not work to remove it. So, the abortionist uses a clamp with sharp teeth to reach inside the woman's vagina, into her cervix, and grasp at the baby's body parts and tear off whatever body part he can reach, pulling it out of the woman's vagina. I once asked an abortion doctor how they decide what to grab first; the answer—they grab whatever is closest.

At twenty-one weeks, the baby is about the size of a small cantaloupe.[103] The baby has feet and toes and is practicing movements like gripping and grabbing the umbilical cord with its hands. The baby can hear as well as differentiate between light and dark. The baby can also taste different foods. A baby girl has a fully formed uterus, and a baby boy has testes producing testosterone.[104] All of its parts must be torn.

The abortionist continues to do this limb by limb, including grasping for the spine, heart, lungs, intestine, and other pieces of the baby's body. Often, the hardest body part to grab and extract is the skull. One abortionist, Dr. Anthony Levatino, explained it this way: "You know you did it right if you crush down on the instrument and white material runs out of the cervix. That was the baby's brain. Then you can pull out skull pieces.... Sometimes a little face comes back and stares at you. Congratulations, you just successfully performed a second trimester D&E abortion."[105]

A curette is used to scrape any remaining parts as well as the placenta. The abortionist then reassembles the baby's body parts on the table because if any part is left behind, the woman will get an infection and could very well die.

Dr. Levatino has testified in court about how he performed over twelve hundred abortions. It wasn't until he saw the death of his own child in his arms that he began to look a little differently at the dead body parts while performing an abortion. He says, "I really looked at that pile of body parts on the side of the table and I didn't see her wonderful right to choose, and I didn't see all of the money I just made, all I could see was somebody's son or daughter."[106]

Is this safe, you may ask? The answer is no. The CDC estimates that the risk of death for a woman undergoing an abortion increases by 38 percent for each additional week of gestation.[107] With every week of pregnancy that passes, larger and sharper fetal bones are being forcibly removed, and they could puncture a woman's uterus or cause a tear in her body. These tears are called perforations and lacerations and can most commonly damage the uterus, cervix, bowel, and bladder. Though it does not happen often, a uterine rupture can cause maternal death.[108]

More likely is increased risk of excessive bleeding and hemorrhaging because the placenta is tightly attached to the lining of the womb at this stage in pregnancy and has been forcibly ripped off. Excessive blood loss can also occur due to injury of the uterus or cervix at this stage. If the cervix does not contract properly after being forcibly opened, a woman can continue bleeding. Scarred cervical tissue is also possible due to the fact that the cervix is forcibly opened so widely to accommodate the removal of a larger child. This can result in other complications like a future miscarriage.[109]

Induction

Abortion by induction is used in the third trimester. Abortion by induction is not at all simple because you are expelling a dead person. In this case, the baby is quite large and cannot be removed via suction or even torn with forceps as I just explained because it is so fully formed. It must be killed inside the womb in order for the procedure to be "successful."

The abortionist uses a large needle to inject digoxin or potassium chloride through the woman's stomach or vagina, typically targeting the baby's heart or head. The abortionist does this so that there is the best chance of killing it right away. Saline and other lethal injections cause the baby's skin to burn over the course of about an hour.[110] No anesthesia is administered to the baby. At a certain point, the lethal dose causes cardiac arrest for the baby, and it will die. If the needle does not hit the baby's heart or head directly, it will still die, but it will take longer. The abortionist may try again to pierce the heart in the hopes he gets it this time. The abortionist will then dilate the woman's cervix. She will go home, with her hopefully dead baby still inside her, and return the next day so the doctor can perform an ultrasound to ensure the baby has died inside the womb.

If the baby appears to be alive, another dose of the lethal injection will be given. The abortionist will then administer labor-inducing drugs. The woman will leave the hospital and go home, while her cervix continues to dilate for about two to four days, so that her cervix can open wide enough to deliver the baby. The woman will return to the clinic to deliver the baby once she is going through severe contractions. If she starts delivering it at home unexpectedly, she will call the abortionist, who will tell her to do it over the toilet. The stillborn will come out then, and she will wait for an abortionist to arrive. If the child does not come out whole, the abortionist will perform a D&E abortion to extract any remaining body parts from the woman.[111] At this point, the baby is roughly a foot to twenty-two inches long.

What I Saw at the Abortion

Richard Selzer, a surgeon attached to Yale University, witnessed an abortion of this nature in 1976, after *Roe v. Wade.* He subsequently wrote about what he witnessed in a series of essays for *Esquire* titled "What I Saw at the Abortion." His *Esquire* essays were honored by the Columbia University Graduate School of Journalism. He was not writing fiction but fact. Selzer had never seen an abortion, even though he worked with surgeons who performed them. One day, he went in with a fellow surgeon as an onlooker. He saw the pregnant woman with a visibly large stomach lay down on the operating table. He saw the abortionist prepare the poisonous injection and prepare to stick it into the stomach of the pregnant woman. Now he's ready. The abortionist "thrusts with his right hand. The needle sinks into the abdominal wall....Another thrust and he has speared the uterus. 'We are in,' he says. Further slight pressure on the needle advances it a bit more....A small geyser of pale yellow fluid erupts. 'We are in the right place,' says the doctor."

Selzer's description is riveting. He continues, "I see something other than what I expected here. I see a movement—a small one. But I have seen it. And then I see it again. And now I see that it is the hub of the needle in the woman's belly that has jerked. First to one side. Then to the other side. Once more it wobbles, is tugged, like a fishing line nibbled by a sunfish....It is the fetus struggling against the needle."

When Selzer pointed to this, the abortionist said it was merely a reflex. The doctor then fed a small tube through the barrel of the needle into the uterus. A pink fluid overran the rim. He withdrew the needle, leaving only the tubing, then attached a syringe with a colorless liquid to the tube and injected it. "Prostaglandin," he said. This was intended to "throw the uterus into vigorous contraction." Over the next eight to twelve hours, the woman would hopefully expel the fetus. If not, time for Round Two. "The doctor detaches the syringe, but does not remove the tubing. 'In case we must do it over,' he says."

Dr. Selzer thought about what he saw—the flick of the needle, it moving back and forth while pierced into the uterus, into the baby in the womb. It was "a defense, a motion from, an effort to get away." He concludes, "For what can language do against the truth of what I saw?"[112]

Abortion Is Unnatural and Not the Same as Childbirth

Many leftists claim that childbirth is just as dangerous as having an abortion. But even if statistically abortion seems to be on the same plane with childbirth, abortion is by definition unnatural. In an abortion procedure, you are intentionally doing something to the woman's body that her body is going to fight you on. All of the ways a woman's body changes during pregnancy are to accommodate the life of the child. Her body is fighting to protect this life. Take something so simple as her placenta attaching to stomach lining. When it is ripped off, she bleeds excessively. Take opening her cervix while it is supporting a fetus. It is going to be difficult to open, and it is unnatural to force it open. Whatever a pregnant woman thinks about abortion, her body knows that it is caring for a little life in there, and the resistance to killing it will be valiant.

Studies show that the risk of depression, anxiety, and suicide are greater for a woman who chooses to abort her baby than for a woman who carries an unwanted pregnancy to term.[113] CBS News reported on a study from the *British Journal of Psychiatry* that looked at whether abortion procedures have a connection with mental health. The study included 877,000 women total, 164,000 of whom had an abortion. The study found that women who had an abortion had an "81 percent increased risk of mental problems."[114] The study also found that the women who got an abortion were "110 percent more likely to abuse alcohol and 155 percent more likely to commit suicide."[115] Interestingly enough, this completely contradicts the pro-choice narrative that "only if women get the abortion they want will they be able to live happy, fulfilled lives." Evidence points to exactly the contrary. It is the women who don't get abortions who are more likely to lead healthy, happy lives.

This is because abortion and childbirth are opposites, one involving a dead child and the other involving a little newborn. When you go through childbirth, you get something out of it. Birth is, of course, an intense process (and thank goodness for the epidural), but at the end of that labor, the mother gets to hold her baby in her arms. When a woman gives birth, a series of happy hormones are released, diminishing the memory of the pain of the experience. The pure joy from a mother holding her baby in her arms for the first time and looking at its little face and hearing its first cry are things that attach the mother to the baby and make the experience worth it. You spent many hours in labor, but now you have this gift that is a part of you and closer to you than anyone else for the rest of your life. Even postpartum depression, which a woman can experience after giving birth, is not a permanent state.

Meanwhile, when you have an abortion, you do not get anything out of it. And you carry the memory with you for the rest of your life. You go through this intense procedure only to hope that you forget it ever happened. You hope to return to normal life, with the dead baby in the container, far behind you. Most women feel deep sadness and regret after aborting a baby. Jennifer O'Neill, American actress and supermodel, said, "I was told a lie from the pit of Hell; that my baby was just a blob of tissue. The aftermath of abortion can be equally deadly for both mother and unborn child. A woman who has an abortion is sentenced to bear that for the rest of her life."[116] O'Neill has since found solace in Jesus Christ and has become a pro-life advocate with *Silence No More*.

Yes, there are women who do not feel an ounce of regret and may even express feelings of happiness having done it. But the only happiness that can come from having an abortion is the sheer relief of not having to do something you did not want to do. The baby is no longer under her sweater, in her pregnant belly, and will never be seen by her again.

The purpose of sharing this information with you, whatever you think about abortion, is to show you that abortion is neither simple nor safe for any of the parties involved.

MY BODY, MY CHOICE

"The only problem is I am not your body"

—FETUS

MYTH: The Constitution guarantees a right to privacy. Abortion is therefore a constitutional right. Abortion is a private decision between a woman and her doctor.

> "*Roe v. Wade* is...a very bad decision. It is bad because it is bad constitutional law, or rather because it is not constitutional law and gives almost no sense of an obligation to try to be."
>
> —JOHN HART ELY, *The Wages of Crying Wolf: A Comment on* ROE V. WADE[117]

Abortion has been recognized as a constitutional right by the Supreme Court since the 1973 landmark case of *Roe v. Wade*. This decision declared that since people have a right to privacy, which the court found to be in the Constitution, a woman has the right to an abortion. Therefore, no state can pass laws, nor can the federal government, to restrict abortion at least before viability. Looking back, it seems absurd that they would highlight the ever-shifting "point of viability," but the Supreme Court did so since it was widely considered to be crucial at the time. Nevertheless, the abortion right is protected today in the United States through the entire nine months of pregnancy. *Roe v. Wade* allowed for some state and federal regulation of abortion, but it is limited. Subsequent decisions interpreting *Roe v. Wade* further narrowed states' ability to regulate abortion.

For those who aren't familiar with the Constitution, it may seem that the document must somewhere mention abortion as a right. But it doesn't. It may also seem that the Constitution invokes some kind of generalized right to privacy that the Supreme Court was able to point to and say, "Here, here is the right to privacy. Privacy is so sacrosanct that it can't be invaded in this case or any other case." But, of course, there's no generalized right to privacy in the Constitution either.

When the Constitution does speak of privacy, it refers to it in particular cases, most notably, unreasonable search and seizure. This means that if you're in your house or you're driving in your car, absent probable cause, the police can't search your house or car without your consent. Why? Because your privacy can't be arbitrarily invaded by the government. But what resemblance does this narrowly specified right to privacy have to an issue like abortion, which does not merely involve the mother but also a father, their unborn child, and her doctor? Clearly the cases are not identical. If the parallel were to work and "right to privacy" were invoked, a woman would have the right to not have her body searched without probable cause. I think that is a fair parallel, and no woman should be subjected to that.

Supreme Court Justice William Rehnquist, who sat on the Court at the time of *Roe v. Wade*, wrote in his dissent that "an operation such as this is not 'private' " and that the right to an abortion is not "even a distant relative" to the justification the Court used, i.e. unreasonable search and seizure, mentioned in the Fourth Amendment.[118]

The Supreme Court went looking elsewhere to find the right to privacy. In its decisions, what the Supreme Court argued, rather strangely, was that the specified right against unreasonable search and seizure, together with other general statements about equal protection of the laws and due process, generate what the court called a penumbra—a kind of emanation or radiation above and beyond what is explicitly said. And supposedly this penumbra protected rights that go beyond the rights actually enumerated in the Constitution.

What we're dealing with here is what the pro-choice side and the Left more generally call "the living constitution." The idea here is that the Constitution itself may be a static document, written by men many years ago, but it can't be interpreted in a static way. Courts are at liberty to use a certain amount of interpretive elasticity to bring the Constitution into line with modern attitudes and modern developments. The Constitution is almost like a living being that grows in accordance with the changing values of the culture. Paul Gewirtz, a professor at Yale Law, agrees with this notion, saying, "The practical content of constitutional principles has surely not been fixed over time but rather has changed as the world changes and the country's moral understandings change."[119]

First of all, no one argues that the Constitution is a purely fixed, static document. The Founders adroitly allowed for a process of change and growth for the Constitution and expected it to occur throughout the nation's future. This process, as you know, is called an "amendment," which can be approved as specified in the Constitution. The passing of an amendment would then presumably change the Constitution to match present-day cultural values. The Founders figured that if values had really changed, then a two-thirds majority would agree on an amendment. If people, through their elected representatives, want the Constitution to be different than it is, they can make it so.

Everyone knows that a two-thirds majority is difficult to get politically, especially on hot-button issues. But this was precisely the intention of the Founders. The Constitution shouldn't be amended every time one side wants something passed for partisan goals because the Constitution is a kind of super law. In a sense, the Constitution overrides the decisions of democratic majorities. It overrides the decisions of states passed through elected state representatives. So to have this kind of super law, the Founders believed there need to be supermajorities of people in the country who want to change the Constitution in this way, who want to make, if you will, a different kind of super law.

This two-thirds majority to amend the Constitution has never been reached regarding abortion. So what you have here in the *Roe v. Wade* decision is judicial usurpation. The justices used the technique or device of interpretation to insert into the Constitution things that it doesn't have and doesn't say. Laurence Tribe, a professor at Harvard Law and a pro-choicer, admits, "One of the most curious things about *Roe* is that, behind its own verbal smokescreen, the substantive judgment on which it rests is nowhere to be found."[120] Pick up a copy of the Constitution. It's not a very thick document. If you hold it up to the light, turn it upside down, squeeze lemon juice on it, doesn't matter, you won't find either a specified right to abortion or even the generalized right to privacy that is so often claimed to be in the Constitution.

Let's think hypothetically about the idea of a right to privacy.

Are we allowed to do anything in the privacy of our own home? We are allowed to do a lot of things, yes, but a few things are off limits. We can't hurt other people, for example. If you are starving your child in your house, protective services will take your child away. If you are abusing your wife, beating her to a pulp, that is not allowed either. Even if there were a "right to privacy," it wouldn't, and shouldn't, justify people killing other people in the privacy of their own home. There is no moral or legal difference, in the sight of the law, between killing in private and killing in public. So why would the right to privacy be invoked here? Because the Supreme Court wanted to reach a certain end result, namely, siding with the right to an abortion rather than a right to life.

Many think that leading up to *Roe v. Wade* there was a grand, larger movement of pro-abortion legislation sweeping the nation. This was not the case and is merely a lie the Left likes to sell in order to justify *Roe v. Wade*. The reality is that the majority of states had pro-life laws and voted to keep them that way. In 1971, just before *Roe v. Wade*, in all twenty-five states that considered legalizing abortion, pro-life legislation prevailed and pro-abortion laws were defeated. In 1972, when Michigan and North Dakota considered on legalizing abortion, both states voted against it in wide margins. Only four liberal states had allowed abortion on demand prior to *Roe v. Wade*.[121]

Roe v. Wade ultimately overturned the laws of all the states that had regulated abortion. And amazingly, the Supreme Court overturned not only the conservative laws prohibiting or severely regulating abortion but also the majority of liberal laws that imposed some, often very minor, constraints on abortion and replaced them with the kind of fiat or decision that in effect said there would be virtually no restriction on abortion. Abortion was now sanctified as a constitutional right placed, you might say, above the reach of the many laws states had passed.

Judge and legal scholar Robert Bork had this to say about *Roe v. Wade*: "When the Court, without warrant in the Constitution, strikes down democratically produced statute, that act substitutes the will of the majority of nine lawyers for the will of the people.... *Roe*, as the greatest example and symbol of the judicial usurpation of democratic prerogatives in this century, should be overturned. The Court's integrity requires that."[122]

When the Constitution protects an enumerated right, say freedom of speech, it then follows that if states or the federal government pass laws restricting speech, those can be struck down on constitutional grounds. But notice that in this case, laws are struck down that regulate a practice that is nowhere mentioned in the Constitution in the name of a right that itself does not exist in the broad, generalized way that it needs to exist for the court to correctly interpret it that way. And when the courts strike down those laws based on this whimsical and arbitrary basis, the net effect is that you the American people do not have the democratic right in your communities, in your localities, in your states, to have laws that reflect the norms of the community in which you live. Even Justice Ruth Bader Ginsburg, who is avidly pro-choice, concedes that *Roe* used "heavy-handed judicial intervention" that was "difficult to justify."[123]

Justice Harry Blackmun, author of the *Roe v. Wade* opinion, famously wrote, "We need not resolve the difficult question of when life begins."[124] If this is true and they did not intend to resolve the "difficult" question of when life begins, why did the court do just that? They decided. And they set a supreme law over the land. If they did not know when life begins, why did they not defer the decision to legislatures? Why did the court choose to prohibit states from voting on this very important issue that has moral weight for many Americans? Michael McConnell, a justice on the United States Court of Appeals for the Tenth Circuit from 2002 to 2009, writes of the court that decided *Roe*, "Worse yet, it was suggesting that the question of human life was irrelevant to the decision."[125]

Not only did the Supreme Court allow nine men to take away from the American people, male and female, the right to make laws, to have democratic control over their own lives on an issue so fundamental as who gets to be a human being, who gets to be allowed into the community, who gets a chance to be born and to live at all, the court also issued a death sentence to millions of children. *Roe v. Wade* was so radically pro-abortion in allowing abortion to the point of birth that it put the United States on par with only a few countries, namely China and North Korea, when it comes to our radical abortion laws.[126]

Roe v. Wade is today sometimes called settled precedent, and it certainly has been around for more than fifty years. Settled precedent is supposed to deserve respect because it is perceived to be anchored in the Constitution and then supported by the practices and customs that have now grown around it and have become part of the body politic.

The reality is that this so-called settled precedent, *Roe v. Wade*, is ultimately based on straw. It is based on constitutional fabrication and reasoning from justices who wanted to bring about a certain outcome. It is a perversion of law, a perversion of true constitutionalism, and ultimately a perversion of the democratic process for them to have done this, leading to the loss of so many lives since 1973, approximately sixty-one million and counting.

Justice Byron White, who sat on the Supreme Court at the time and voted against *Roe v. Wade*, wrote in his dissent, "I find nothing in the language or history of the Constitution to support the Court's judgment. The Court simply fashions a new constitutional right."[127] He pointedly called this decision "an exercise of raw judicial power."[128]

More recently, Alan Dershowitz, lawyer and professor at Harvard Law, in an interview with *Business Insider* said, "I support a woman's right to choose, I always have."[129] Yet even he recognizes that *"Roe v. Wade* was a disaster" and argues that it was not constitutional.

Ultimately, *Roe v. Wade* will go down in history as one of the most constitutionally baseless and wicked decisions of the Supreme Court, one comparable to the *Plessy v. Ferguson* decision that enshrined segregation or the *Dred Scott v. Sanford* decision, which ultimately said that black people have no rights that whites are to respect. These decisions were overturned and tossed onto the ash heap of history. This should be the fate of *Roe v. Wade*. And the sooner the better.

CHAPTER SIX

MYTH: Poor women need access to abortion. In order for something to be a right, it must be meaningfully exercised. Abortion must be taxpayer funded.

"The idea of rights is nothing but the conception of virtue applied to the world of politics."[130]

—ALEXIS DE TOCQUEVILLE

In the three years following the *Roe v. Wade* decision, the federal government paid for abortions through Medicaid, covering about 300,000 abortion procedures each year. In 1974, this payment accounted for roughly one-third of all abortions nationwide. The burden placed on taxpayers was about $55 million per year.[131] To much of the public, this was a bridge too far—being forced to pay for something as morally objectionable as abortions. A champion of this position emerged in the person of Illinois congressman Henry Hyde. He knew that he could not undo what the Supreme Court had ruled, and he knew that abortion had been codified as constitutional. He also knew that it was a completely different story to ask the public to pay for something so morally repugnant. His energetic efforts were to become a beacon of hope for the anti-abortion forces.

Representative Hyde sought to prevent the federal government from using taxpayers' money to bankroll abortion operations across the country. The Hyde Amendment, as it came to be known, does just that. It prohibits federal money from being used to fund abortions. It protects most Americans from being forced to pay for an abortion that is not their own. In doing this, it also protects religious liberty as well as freedom of conscience. However, individual states could still fund abortions, and about sixteen states have done so. In those states, taxpayers do pay for women to get abortions.

But if you don't live in one of those sixteen states, by and large, the individual has to pay for her own abortion. This is what the pro-abortion movement wants to change. The Left's argument for federal funding of abortion is that abortion is a constitutional right in the same way that free speech is a right or freedom of religion is a right. Thus, the pro-choicer would argue that if something is a basic right and you can't afford it, then the government should provide it to you. What is the point of having a right that cannot be exercised?

So, the pro-abortion argument goes, is it fair to deprive poor women of their constitutional right to abortion? This argument at first glance might seem to make sense, but upon reflection, it collapses. Let's consider our basic rights. We have a First Amendment right to free speech. But ask yourself, is that funded by the government? If I can't afford a newspaper or Internet, will the government pay for that for me? No. I have a First Amendment right to freedom of religion. Will the government build me a church if my friends and I can't afford to put one up? No. I have a Second Amendment right to own a gun. Will the government buy me the gun and the ammunition? No. So down the list of rights we go, and it becomes clear that none of our fundamental rights are paid for by the government.

In practice, these rights are essentially protections against the government. If you think about the Bill of Rights, its formulations go something like this: Congress shall make no law restricting freedom of speech. Congress shall make no law restricting freedom of religion. The idea here is that the government is a threat to rights, and by placing limitations on government power, your rights are protected. Interestingly, with abortion, the Left wants to go in the other direction. They want to empower the government and want the government to have a bigger role—quite the opposite from limiting the government. By demanding that abortion is a right that must be funded, when our other fundamental rights are not, the Left is saying that they want abortion to be a super right. One may say that in the church of modern liberalism, abortion has become a sacrament.

Even if you think the government should pay for some aspect of health care, abortion is not a right, and it certainly is not health care. Abortion is killing.

For nearly forty years, the Hyde Amendment has been an effective obstacle to the pro-abortion agenda. We must protect Hyde and vote for politicians who support it because even mainstream Democrats are ready to take it down. Federal funds currently go to Planned Parenthood, not for abortion but for the other services it provides. But obviously, the federal funding given to it to cover its other costs allows it to continue its wholesale abortion operations. This is why beyond protecting the Hyde Amendment, we must vote to defund Planned Parenthood. There are other worthy women's health organizations that actually provide health care to women that do not involve killing babies. I will say more about Planned Parenthood in a later chapter.

The Radicalization of the Democrats

America has profoundly changed since 1973 when *Roe v. Wade* was decided. The Supreme Court decision was so radically pro-abortion that it didn't even match the tide of the country at the time. Three years after *Roe v. Wade*, the Hyde Amendment was passed by the majority of Democrats, who controlled the House at the time. More than a hundred Democrats voted in favor of Hyde, providing more than half of the support for the bill. That same year, both presidential nominees—Jimmy Carter and Ronald Reagan—opposed abortion. Later, both Presidents Bill Clinton and Barack Obama endorsed the Hyde Amendment.

But times have changed. Every candidate in the 2020 race for the Democratic nomination for president was anti–Hyde Amendment. Bernie Sanders tweeted, "There is #NoMiddle Ground on women's rights. Abortion is a constitutional right. Under my Medicare for All Plan, we will repeal the Hyde Amendment."[132] Elizabeth Warren tweeted, "It's time for Hyde to go."[133] Kirsten Gillibrand tweeted, "Repealing the Hyde Amendment is critical."[134] Cory Booker tweeted, "The Hyde Amendment is a threat to reproductive rights."[135] Pete Buttigieg echoed this when he told his supporters that we are all "lifted up" by stories about abortion and that his health care plan would "support, reimburse, and fund" abortion.[136]

In all the strident pro-abortion squalling among "progressive" Democrats, former vice president Joe Biden was most uncomfortable as he continued his forty-year tap dance on the abortion issue. He consistently voted for the Hyde Amendment throughout his Senate career, and in 1981 Biden supported a constitutional amendment that would enable the overturning of *Roe v. Wade*. In his 2007 book *Promises to Keep*, he wrote that he was "personally opposed" to abortion but that he didn't have the "right to impose" his view on the rest of society. He stated that he wouldn't support federal funding of abortion but that he was all of a sudden against a constitutional amendment to limit abortion. Now, he says he believes that abortion should be funded by taxpayers and describes it as "healthcare" and "a right."[137]

It is increasingly clear that many Democratic politicians are either ideologues devoted to furthering the radical Left's agenda, like Bernie Sanders, or simply hungry for power and change their positions in order to be the most popular, like Joe Biden. In any case, over the past several years, there has been a radicalization of the Democratic Party.

While the Democrats have not been able to take down the Hyde Amendment, they are trying their best to do so. If they take over the presidency, keep control of the House, and take the Senate, the Hyde Amendment is history. It might seem that the pro-choice movement would be content with abortion on demand, but no, the Democrats are pushing for abortion to be federally funded by you and me.

Ironically, the Hyde Amendment has been upheld by the Supreme Court. In the 1980 decision *Harris v. McRae*, the court held that Hyde did not contradict the Constitution and that states with Medicaid were not obligated to fund abortions. The American Center for Law and Justice says that "abortion advocates constantly argue that abortion is a decision between a woman and her doctor. Yet if the Hyde Amendment is repealed, every American will become involved in abortions through the use of our tax dollars.

For those of us who believe life is precious no matter the circumstances, the consequences are dire."[138]

Most Americans do not agree with the Democrats on this issue. A 2019 Marist poll found that only 39 percent of Americans supported taxpayer dollars funding abortion.[139] Ultimately, it doesn't make sense how someone else's choices are zero percent my business and at the same time 100 percent my fiscal responsibility.

CHAPTER SEVEN

MYTH: Women have the freedom to choose what they want to do with their body—when to have children and with whom.

"The only freedom which deserves the name is that of pursuing our own good in our own way, so long as we do not attempt to deprive others of theirs, or impede their efforts to obtain it."

—JOHN STUART MILL, *On Liberty*[140]

Consider this personal account that appeared in *Slate* magazine: "I just recall riding in my friend's convertible VW Bug, and the top was down. Us in the car with our hair flying everywhere, which felt like a romantic young moment of freedom and abandon, but we're going to go get one of us an abortion." The woman, Anna Holmes, founder of the blog Jezebel, described her feelings after aborting her baby: "I just recall getting back in the VW Bug with the top down and driving back to my hometown about 15 miles away, with the hair flying everywhere, all of us."[141]

This may seem like a scene out of Jack Kerouac's novel *On the Road*, with the image of freedom, the open road, and the wind in her hair, but it was about a trip to an abortion clinic. To Anna Holmes, abortion is the pure expression of freedom, and choice is expressed as a moral ideal. She says she has had three abortions so far (one at eighteen, one around twenty-two, one at twenty-seven), and she seems to relish the memories of her abortion experiences. She says of her abortions, "I did feel a certain amount of pride in the fact that I was living my principles. I'd grown up pro-choice, I had gone to pro-choice rallies with my mother when I was a kid in San Francisco. But being pro-choice in theory and being pro-choice in action... I just felt like I lived my stated principles, that my body was mine to control, that women's bodies are theirs to control. I never felt guilty about it."[142]

For the pro-choice movement, choice is the value upon which everything else resides. Choice is the word they use most often. The power of using the word "choice" is that it appeals to the idea of freedom. Freedom is one of the core values of the West, and it's one of the core values that most of us uphold. We see the American Revolution as a struggle for freedom from the British, giving us the right to rule ourselves. Our individuality is the expression of our freedom of our choices; they are what make us who we are. And all of this, this appeal to freedom, and to choice, is being invoked to justify something as clinical, as harmful, and as terrible as the mass killing of unborn human beings. So how do we confront this most devious justification for abortion in the name of freedom itself? The choice they are referring to, after all, is not "the idea of choice" in general. They are referring to the choice to do something specific: the choice to kill.

If I had to pick a single mantra we hear most often from pro-choicers today, it is "my body, my choice." Pro-choicers try to muddy the waters by making it out as though the woman is exercising power and exercising choice over *her body alone*. But is it only "her body" she is referring to? Is it her body she wants to abort? Of course not. How would one abort oneself? We all know that, actually, it is not "her body" she is referring to but the fetus's body.

But in order for the Left to pull off the argument that the fetus is literally "her body," as they claim, they must argue that the fetus is a body part that can be removed, just like her appendix or her tonsils. Imagine how ridiculous this is since we know the fetus is not a body part but a living being with its own heartbeat and body parts. As I have shown, no matter what developmental stage the fetus is in, it is at no point "an organ." Organs are body parts that enable us to function. Her heart is pumping blood, her lungs are helping her to breathe, her brain is enabling her mind to function, and so on. The "my body, my choice" argument breaks down when we realize that during pregnancy, when the woman is "with child," there are two sets of body parts—mother and child. The fetus is inside her body temporarily during the nine months of pregnancy, but it is not "her body."

Let's turn to the issue of choice. We have a whole movement that calls itself not the "pro-abortion movement" but "the pro-choice movement." And pro-choice, on the face of it, is basically the notion that choices are good and choices should be wide open. People should be able to make their own choices, the argument goes, particularly on something as important as pregnancy. No one would disagree that we all want choices in life. We seek choices. We measure our level of responsibility by the choices we make.

The ultimate champion of choice, and champion of freedom, is the philosopher John Stuart Mill. He articulates these ideas in his work *On Liberty*. As one of the fathers of libertarianism, he lays out the doctrine of limited government and maximal individual freedom. There's a wise libertarian suspicion of the government intervening in choices that are within our legitimate purview or domain. And I think this skepticism of government makes sense because most things are better resolved by the local community and individual. It seems, then, that Mill's argument would fall on the pro-choice side. But not so.

He says, "No one pretends that actions should be as free as opinions."[143] To limit the mind is to limit individuality and uniqueness, so it should never be limited. However, he finds that there is a limit to freedom of action; it can never be absolute.

The central tenet of libertarianism states that my right to swing my arm only extends as far as your face. In other words, my rights stop when they begin to harm or affect others. So freedom is paramount, but to a point. Why to a point? Because harming someone or killing them is to take away that person's freedom. You can't in the very name of freedom take away another's freedom.

So while the government should stay out of most things in order to allow for maximum individual freedom, a true libertarian would have to agree that if there's one thing the government must stop, it is the killing of other innocent people and the robbing of their freedom. Rand Paul, one of the most outspoken libertarians today, says, "I am 100 percent pro-life."[144]

Abortion comes to the forefront of our minds when we think of the fact that legally today in America, people can be killed at whim, their freedom and future, obliterated. It seems like we wouldn't be able to think of a similar scenario, where the side that strangely advocates for a horror such as this calls themselves "pro-choice." But when we think about American history, we find a parallel that is almost identical to the abortion debate today. And that is the debates that ensued over slavery leading up to the Civil War. If we look at the Lincoln-Douglas debates, the famous debates in the middle of the nineteenth century between two statesmen, Abraham Lincoln and Stephen Douglas, we see that their debates are very similar in substance and, in fact, almost identical in form to the abortion debate.[145]

Both of them were running for the Senate in Illinois, a preview of their presidential campaigns against each other four years later. Lincoln was the Republican; Douglas was the Democrat. And they were debating, of course, not abortion but slavery.

Here's Stephen Douglas arguing that he is for choice. In fact, he says he's neither for slavery nor against it. He says that he doesn't care if slavery is voted up or down. The point he wants to make is that we live in a big country. Some people, he says, are for slavery, some people are anti-slavery. Douglas says it seems unreasonable to take one of these positions, a single norm you might say, and impose that set of values on the whole country. He says, rather, why not adopt a democratic solution? Why don't we agree to disagree? Why don't we embrace the principle of choice? So, Douglas advocates what he calls "popular sovereignty."

But what he means by popular sovereignty is really what we today call the pro-choice position. He says let every community, every territory, every state decide for itself if it wants slavery. And in this way, Douglas says, we're able to have a society in which different sets of values can coexist. By affirming the pro-choice position, Douglas says, we have a framework that is very consistent with the core principle of America and of the Founders: the principle of freedom. This, you can see, is a very attractive argument, and it's not immediately obvious how it can be rebutted. It sounds good!

Let's now consider Lincoln's refutation of Douglas because

Lincoln makes, I think, one of the strongest arguments not just against slavery but, as it turns out, for the pro-life position as well. And Lincoln basically says choice is a good thing, but choice always depends on what it is that is being chosen. Lincoln says, if the black man is like a hog, then, sure, it makes sense to choose whether you want to buy or sell it. But on the other hand, if the Negro is a human being, that same argument now collapses. But why does it collapse? What is the difference between a human being and a hog? For Lincoln, the difference is this: we do not, as human beings, have the right to use choice to deny others their life choices. We don't have the right to use our choice to cancel out the choices of other people.

And this argument applies with equal force to slavery and abortion. We don't have the right to choose to enslave others, and neither do we have the right to choose to kill them. If we do claim this right, the right to enslave or the right to kill, Lincoln argues that what we're embracing is the right of the powerful to exploit the vulnerable. And what is particularly sickening is that this exploitation is then masked in the language of freedom. Lincoln very poignantly says that the wolf and the sheep both use the language of freedom, but they mean two different things by it. For the wolf, the freedom is the freedom to eat the sheep. For the sheep, freedom is the freedom to be free of the wolf, the freedom to live as a sheep.

To quote Lincoln, "The shepherd drives the wolf from the sheep, for which the sheep thanks the shepherd as his Liberator, while the wolf denounces him for the same act as the destroyer of liberty." "Plainly," says Lincoln sarcastically, "the sheep and the wolf are not agreed upon a definition of liberty."[146] The most noble interpretation of choice is a choice to affirm life, not to degrade it, not to enslave it, not to wantonly take it.

Betsey DeVos, secretary of education, talked about the similarities between slavery and abortion in a lecture she gave at Colorado Christian University. DeVos invoked Lincoln and said, "He too contended with the 'pro-choice' arguments of his day." She continued, "Lincoln was right about the slavery 'choice' then, and he would be right about the life 'choice' today."[147]

Most pro-choicers go into the mode of denial when discussing "the choice to kill," claiming abortion isn't killing and there's no death involved. It's refreshing to hear an honest response from a pro-choice feminist like Naomi Wolf, who admits that abortion involves a death and even requires mourning. In her essay "Our Bodies, Our Souls," she warns that the pro-choice movement needs to stop its denial and acknowledge the deaths of babies, or it risks becoming "precisely what our critics charge us with being: callous, selfish and casually destructive men and women who share a cheapened view of human life." She believes that the pro-choice Left is "in danger of losing something more important than votes; we stand in jeopardy of losing our souls."

One might expect that this realization would lead her to back away from pro-choice ideology, but alas it only leads her to argue that the pro-choice movement's problem isn't its ideology but its marketing. She finds the pro-choice language of describing abortion as "between a woman and her doctor" too clinical and believes it has led to "political failure." Instead she says it should be described as "between a woman and God." That sounds better, and more heartfelt, potentially endearing more people to the pro-choice side. She says to pro-choicers, by "using amoral rhetoric, we weaken ourselves politically."[148] She credits the pro-life side for tapping into morality and thinks pro-choicers should use the language of God more, too.

Ultimately, "pro-choice" is a contradiction in terms because it is a choice to cancel out the choices of people who have not even had a chance to make any choices in the world at all. Pro-choice is ultimately a moral abomination and a moral degradation. Phrasing it as "a choice between you and God" is a cop-out that doesn't really work because every decision we make in life is between the self and God, and the fact that one is accountable to God for this choice is no exception. Regardless of personal belief in God and God's judgment, the taking of an innocent life is a case where the government should intervene. Why? Because it is the core function of government to protect our right to life, upon which all other rights flow. The right to life, liberty, and the pursuit of happiness, as outlined in the Declaration of Independence, is powerful. But if you take my life, you also take my liberty and my chance at happiness.

CHAPTER EIGHT

MYTH: Men do not belong in the abortion debate. This is a women's issue.

"It takes two to tango."

—*Old saying*

Brad Allen, living in Nebraska in 2019, was distraught when the mother of his unborn son, Liam, insisted upon having an abortion against his wishes. "I put up every legal and sane roadblock to save my child's life,"[149] says Allen. But there was nothing he could do to stop the abortion. Allen had no right to see the pre-abortion ultrasound or to view the remains of his son. Perhaps worst of all, he was denied any official verification that the procedure had taken place and that his child was dead. What had happened in Brad Allen's case was perfectly legal. The Supreme Court ruled in *Planned Parenthood v. Casey* that "spousal awareness," having women notify the father of an abortion, was an undue burden on the woman and, therefore, unconstitutional. Any state laws requiring that a woman notify the father of her baby were struck down by this Supreme Court ruling.

In Brad Allen's case, he felt a deep sense of loss after Liam's death and sought healing through counseling. He describes the first step in the healing process as "denial," and in order to move past denial, he was told that he must face the truth in order to grieve and move on. "About a month after Liam's abortion," Allen explained, "I wanted to honor my son's life with an obituary in the *Omaha World Herald*." But the paper refused to print the obituary without a death certificate. Allen then sought to obtain a death certificate. He knew that Nebraska law allowed death certificates to be issued for babies who died during miscarriage. But Allen was in for an astounding surprise; Nebraska law prohibits issuing death certificates for babies who are "intentionally demised." Allen's reaction was one of despair and confusion. He says, "The justifications for the certificate law were to give dignity to the lost life and help grieving families heal. This begged the question, why can't aborted babies receive the same dignity? Aren't post-abortion parents in need of healing too?"

Allen then joined forces with Dr. Pat Castle of a group called LIFE Runners. They recruited a coalition of Nebraska postabortion counselors to show that there were other parents, who lost a child in abortion, who were also in need of some way to cope and begin the healing process with an official death certificate acknowledging the death of their child—just as parents who have lost a child in miscarriage do. Postabortion mother and counselor Jeannie Pittman was granted a death certificate for her daughter, Grace. She had finagled it through an organization called Vital Records that was acting as a sort of "underground railroad," helping families in need of healing obtain death certificates from state records for abortions. Finally, Allen got Liam's death certificate on December 5, 2019, in Lincoln, Nebraska. What he learned there on the cold, official statement was that his son had been dismembered by notorious abortionist LeRoy Carhart and that his remains were discarded as medical waste. But as awful as it was to see these words, at least he now had an official account of Liam's death.

In an article Allen later recalled, "The moment I was handed the certificate I felt an immense wave of healing. My aborted baby had just taken a step toward personhood and been elevated to the same status of a miscarried baby." Allen views the documentation of Liam's dismemberment as a historic step and sees Liam as a part of the "state-documented victims of this holocaust that is abortion."

Pro-choice advocates frame abortion as a "women's issue." Since it's the woman's body, it's the woman's choice. Men have no place in the abortion debate. You'll see signs at the Women's March that say "No Uterus, No Opinion." But the people who say that don't mean it strictly. They're actually happy to have men along with women in the demonstration lines or in rallies championing the pro-choice cause, but they are very angry when they see men, or women for that matter, on the pro-life side. More importantly, they don't want the man who is the father of the child to have any meaningful say in the fate of his child. The woman might consult the man if she wants to, but she isn't under any obligation to do so. It's her decision alone.

When the mother calls into question the very life and death of their child, does it make sense for the father to be left in the dark? In this witch's brew of confusion, let's consider the irrefutable facts. When a child is conceived, a mother and a father took part in making this child. This child is a combination of both of them, bearing half the DNA of the mother and half the DNA of the father. Yet the baby is its own entity, a unique being that will never exist again. So, who is the owner of this entity?

Let's look at an entirely different scenario, not involving abortion but involving who has ownership over frozen embryos. John Terrell and Ruby Torres were dating in 2014, and upon finding out that Ruby had cancer but before undergoing chemotherapy, Ruby began in vitro fertilization using John Terrell as a sperm donor. The couple signed a contract with the fertility clinic stating that any fertilized eggs were joint property and "both parties would have to agree about what to do with them if the relationship ended," according to an NBC report.150 The couple married and divorced without any children. The frozen embryos remained frozen, so to speak.

After the breakup, Ruby decided that she wanted to use the frozen embryos that she had created with Terrell before they were married. She claimed that she could not create new frozen embryos with another sperm donor now, since she had undergone chemotherapy. A lower court in Arizona ruled that the woman's desire to become pregnant "outweighed" the man's desire to not become a father, and the court ruled in favor of Ruby Torres. In 2018, the state of Arizona established a law allowing women to use frozen embryos without the father's consent. But the provision was not retroactive, meaning the case between Terrell and Torres, dating back to 2014, should be decided based on their contract. This case was appealed and went all the way to the Arizona Supreme Court, and their contract was upheld. Their contract required "written consent" from both parties, and Terrell would not provide that consent.

The point here is that outside of the abortion debate there is an equally passionate debate over the ownership of an embryo. It is not clear whether the woman or the man should have free rein over it. If it was clearly the "body of the woman," then there would have never been a legal battle over the embryo in the first place. Clearly the embryo is its own entity. But the argument that men have absolutely nothing to do with the embryo is scientifically wrong because any fertilized embryo is 50 percent the man and 50 percent the woman.

The argument that abortion is exclusively a women's rights issue conflicts with a much larger movement in our society—the growing effort to involve men more in tasks that take place in the home. Early feminism contested the distinction between stereotypically women's tasks and men's tasks, deriding "the cult of domesticity." For example, men would focus on providing for the family through work outside the home, and women would either stay home or, perhaps, work a steady job with fewer hours and less pay. But the man would be the main provider, and the woman would be in charge of keeping the home in order and raising the children. This was the case about seventy years ago and is how we often stereotypically view the 1950s American family.

But much has changed since then. While some families operate in this fashion, others operate in a manner quite different. What has changed is societal expectations of men and women. Many families decide for themselves how to run their family unit, and that can be done in a variety of ways. Overall, men and women are beginning to share household tasks as well as the care of children. (Of course, there are also families where both parents work full-time outside the home, so it is actually a nanny or another third party who does the majority of the child-rearing.)

Whatever we think of this shift, it is clearly happening. The fact that both parents are expected to be involved in children's lives—financially, emotionally, and physically—means that excluding one parent entirely from the process and saying that "it's not their issue to care about" does not align with the times.

A pro-choice leftist would argue that it's the woman who has to carry the baby for nine months, so even if the man wants to raise the child and is willing to help out during her pregnancy, he'll never experience what she's going through. Of course he isn't birthing the baby, but is this characterization really true? Good fathers are very often at the woman's beck and call during the pregnancy. They not only help during this time but in some cases go through physical symptoms that mirror the woman's, showing that there is actually a kind of link between the man, woman, and child in this experience.

What impact does abortion have on the man? One can only imagine that men are affected by losing a child, in some cases affected deeply or even traumatized by it. In an article by the BBC, the focus is on an Alabama case where a man tells a news agency that he tried to plead with the mother of his child. "I just tried to plead with her...talk to her about it and see what I could do. But in the end, there was nothing I could do to change her mind." She went ahead with the abortion anyway.

Another fellow, Karl Locker, says that when he was in his thirties, he was living the single life, and he made a woman pregnant. When he found out about it, he was "like one of those wolves with its legs caught in a trap," he explains. Then when he thought about it, he realized he had to support her and the pregnancy. "I tried everything. I offered to marry her, to take the baby myself, or to offer it up for adoption." The woman said she could never give her child up for adoption. But ironically, she didn't mind having it aborted. Mr. Locker adds that even though he ended up paying for the abortion, it had a traumatic effect on him. "I didn't know how I was going to survive; I wasn't going to jump off a bridge, but I probably would have drunk myself to death.... I've thought about what happened every day for the last 32 years."

Another man, Chuck Raymond, whose eighteen-year-old girl-friend had an abortion in the late 1970s, said that at the time he was in military training at West Point. He says that he suppressed what happened for many years. But years later, he says, "I realized the tragedy that had occurred and that we had made a tragic choice." He likens the mental and emotional anguish that follows abortion to the kind of PTSD that one might get after being on a battlefield. He has been haunted for years.[151]

These kinds of voices are excluded from the abortion debate. The pro-choice side clearly doesn't care about how the woman's choice affects the man who is the father. While the Left acts as though they appreciate "men expressing their feelings" in other circumstances and encourage men to be "vulnerable," they don't actually want to hear what breaks the hearts of men the most.

Mostly when men are referenced in this debate, they're referenced in a negative context. Here is Sarah Wheat, who works for Planned Parenthood in Austin: "Outside our clinics, it's typically men who are leading the protests and clambering onto cars to yell over the fence with bull horns."[152] The Left loves to paint the pro-life movement as one led by men, but this is actually completely false because if you look at the leaders of pro-life organizations, they are mostly women. Look at Alveda King, niece of Martin Luther King Jr., who has been an advocate for civil rights for the unborn, or Marjorie Dannenfelser, president of the Susan B. Anthony List, or Lila Rose, founder and president of the organization Live Action, or Jeanne Mancini, president of the March for Life. Kind, strong, intelligent, fearless women are in the forefront of pro-life activism.

But nevertheless, the Left is desperate to create a caricature of the angry man who just wants to control women's bodies. Why don't they show pictures of Catholic nuns marching peacefully quoting Mother Teresa's pro-life sayings like "Give the child to me" or the teenage girls whose signs say, "My mom walked out of the abortion clinic and chose life," or the mom whose sign says, "My cluster of cells is now a student at Stanford," or all of the women who march and say, "Love them both." Love the woman and love the baby. The pro-life movement is made up of a lot of women, of all ages, and couldn't be more genuine and loving as well as men who could not be more supportive, but that is exactly what irritates the Left so much.

Why does the Left create this image of angry men? Because they want this issue to become a battle of the sexes, where it's the free, brave, pro-choice woman on the one side and the evil, controlling, anti-abortion man on the other. Ironically, I see far more angry people at leftist protests than any pro-life event I have ever been to. Most pro-choicers that go to the Women's March, for example, are wearing Pussyhats, carrying signs that say "F**k Trump," and screaming at people.

What we can learn from how the Left uses this imagery to portray this issue is that it reflects their way of thinking. They will stop at nothing to justify abortion on demand. And they will continue to package it and sell it however they can in order to achieve their goals. Meanwhile, we must stay focused on truth and advocate for all parties involved. At the end of the day, the woman is deeply affected by abortion, and the man is deeply affected by abortion. But the person who is affected more than anyone is the child who is brutally dismembered, as was Brad Allen's son Liam in Nebraska.

Just as motherhood begins in the womb, fatherhood begins in the womb. We must acknowledge the important fact that some fathers are willing to raise their child even if the woman isn't. And yet they are never taken into consideration and are not given any rights under the law. This is an abomination and frankly a deep disservice to both father and child. Shouldn't the child's best interest be considered by the government? Why can't the child's own father who wants to raise it do so? This should not be a controversial idea. Dads should be empowered to raise their kids, and the media should celebrate dads who do so. I think it would be a beautiful solution to a difficult situation to have a woman who was going to get an abortion instead give the child to the father who wants to raise it. Wouldn't the child be better off left in the arms of its father than at the hands of the abortionist? What the mother might call her choice the father could call his son or his daughter.

A POSITIVE GOOD

"Woe to those who call evil good and good evil."

—ISAIAH 5:20

MYTH: Abortion is necessary in order for women to fully control their own bodies. Without abortion, women don't have reproductive freedom or equality. Since men do not have to live with consequences of free sex, women shouldn't have to either.

"What a piece of work is a man! How noble in reason, how infinite in faculty! In form and moving how express and admirable! In action how like an angel, in apprehension how like a god! The beauty of the world. The paragon of animals."[153]

—WILLIAM SHAKESPEARE, *Hamlet*

While "choice" is important to some left-wingers, others emphasize the power of abortion itself. Abortion is a good thing, they say. Left-wing author Katha Pollitt writes, "The framing of abortion as reproductive justice rather than simple choice is important."[154] One of the most remarkable arguments of the pro-abortion advocates is that abortion promotes reproductive equality for women. Without abortion, the pro-abortion activists say, women don't have reproductive freedom or equality with men. Since men don't have to live with the consequences of free sex, women shouldn't have to either.

The pro-abortion activists ask—Are you trying to take us back to puritanical times before the Sexual Revolution, when women had virtually no control over their own bodies and over their own pregnancies? If women are forced to birth children, we hear, they won't be able to finish school, will have to take maternity leave, and will be left behind in the workplace. They will face unfair social stigma for being a mother. We hear that abortion produces greater equality between the sexes because it enables women to control their own bodies.

Is Abortion Necessary for Women to Control Their Own Bodies?

First, is it really true that without abortion women can't control their bodies? Left-wing feminists argue that abortion is like contraception in that both are a means for women to control their bodies. This is incredibly misleading and factually untrue. Most of the time hormonal birth control creates an environment that prevents fertilization from occurring the first place, but there are rare times depending on the type of birth control when a fertilized egg is prevented from being implanted. However, this is never the case for barrier methods of contraception. In these cases, of course, abortion is nothing like contraception. Scientifically, barrier contraception devices—be that a male condom diaphragm, cervical cap, or contraceptive sponge—prevent pregnancy from occurring in the first place. While barrier contraception works to prevent pregnancy from occurring in the first place, abortion terminates a pregnancy. Those two things, far from being the same, are in fact opposites. Left-wing feminists lump contraception and abortion together as "reproductive health," acting as if they are a package deal. In fact, because men and women have access to contraception, we should not need abortion.

There's also natural family planning, which is limiting your sexual activity to times of the month when you are less fertile. Condoms are 98 percent effective, but even taking into account user error, which renders them typically 85 percent effective, if you combine natural family planning with using a condom, your chances of getting pregnant are even lower than your chance of being in a plane crash. Couples can have 99.99 percent control over their bodies in terms of pregnancy if precautionary measures are taken. While natural family planning and condoms can be used if you don't want to have a child at this time in life but may want to later, there are other means of preventing pregnancy if you never want to have children, like a vasectomy, hysterectomy, or tubal ligation. Never in the history of the world have there been so many convenient ways to avoid becoming pregnant. And that, it would seem, is the ultimate control a woman has over her body. With this sort of control, there is simply no reason why abortion should be used as a form of birth control.

Our culture pits sexuality and the family against each other. Through the media, the culture conveys the message that having casual sex is the definition of living a single and free lifestyle, while being married and having children is the definition of a sexless lifestyle, when in fact, it is and should be the opposite. Having children and being married inherently involves sex, and this makes sense. When sex is freely exercised in marriage, problems like abortion for reasons other than to preserve the life of the mother rarely arise. The beauty of fun, frequent sex in marriage is an idea the Leftist culture we live in vehemently opposes because it thwarts their goal to promote casual sex. To the Left, sex outside marriage should be the norm. But what the Left leaves out is that this casual sex culture leads to the breakdown of the family, the source of many other problems.

Why Can't a Woman Be More Like a Man?

Consider now the broader topic raised by this debate on equality. In *My Fair Lady*, Henry Higgins sarcastically quips, "Why can't a woman be more like a man?" Feminists on the Left, however, take the idea very seriously. They often say, "Even with birth control, the genders aren't equal. Why doesn't the man have to carry the pregnancy? Why doesn't he have the big belly showing everyone that he's pregnant? The man has it easier than the woman."

The attorneys in *Abramowicz v. Lefkowitz*, a 1969 case before *Roe v. Wade*, drew attention to the clear discrepancy between men and women in order to argue in favor of abortion rights for women. The attorneys claimed that "the man who shares responsibility for her pregnancy can and often does just walk away."[155] The attorneys argued that women must enjoy that same freedom—to walk away. Abortion, they argued, is the necessary answer, so that woman can enjoy full equality on par with the man in this respect.

So, as you can see, rather than calling upon men to step up to the plate, the Left decided that it is better to let both parties off the hook. Both parties being able to engage in free sex without consequence is the highest value here, and being able to walk away from an unforeseen outcome must be the gold standard. The Left sort of expects men to not step up and expects women to just get an abortion. How horrible is this? The prevalence of abortion in the country has made both parties perhaps more "equal" in a weird sense, but only by leveling them to a lower playing field, free of responsibility.

Gloria Steinem, the leader of the left-wing feminist movement that is tied to abortion, coined the term "reproductive freedom." In 2013, President Barack Obama awarded Steinem the Presidential Medal of Freedom, the highest honor that can be awarded to civilians in the United States.[156] Referring to gender equality, she told *Variety* in 2020, "If we did not have wombs, we'd be fine."[157]

Unfortunately, many women who follow the left-wing feminist ideology of Gloria Steinem are constantly waging war on the female body while acting like men are the greatest. In her article "If Men Could Menstruate," Steinem says that if men had periods, "menstruation would become an enviable, worthy, masculine event."[158] But this shows that she underlyingly thinks that men have the upper hand just by virtue of having better minds than us, of framing the same situation in a better way. They're more positive. They're go-getters. They make lemonade out of lemons.

But I don't like this attitude. Women are plenty good at making lemonade out of lemons, and I certainly do not even agree with her assumption because I think if men got a period, or something like it in an alternate universe, they would probably get used to it and learn to live with it, as women do and as humans do with most bodily functions. They'd probably hate that time of the month like we do.

The feminist Shulamith Firestone famously describes the fetus as "the uninvited guest." Political essayist Ellen Willis echoes this notion by describing abortion as "an act of self-defense."[159] Firestone even goes so far as to say that "pregnancy is barbaric."[160] Not only does this ideology purport that babies are intruders, but it also implies that women's bodies are inherently treacherous for housing these intruders. Since pregnancy is unique to women, it creates a feeling of self-loathing for the woman who believes this warped ideology. If the standard of greatness is literally "being a man," women will inherently never meet that standard. The female body, pre- or post-motherhood as well as during pregnancy, should be accepted and celebrated.

Women often fall into the trap of thinking that "we have to be like men in order to be powerful. Whatever a man does, I'm going to do." And to a certain point that makes sense. Since men were traditionally the ones coming up with the great inventions, the great books, the great ideas, aspiring to do those things is what women should strive for, not because men do them but because they are inherently great ambitions in and of themselves. But there are also inherently beautiful things about being a woman, and there are tangible benefits to being a woman in many situations as well.

But do men really have it better? Take their inherent strength. What are the consequences of men being stronger? Well, when there are dangerous tasks, like going into a mine, fighting in a war, or being drafted, then men are called upon to serve first. The superior strength of the man is taken as a starting point because social demands are placed on men that are not automatically placed on women. To this day, if a family is attacked by a marauder or an outsider, the man is expected to be the one to take the lead in fighting back, to risk his life for the women and children.

As for the downside of being a woman, let's start with pregnancy since that is framed as the bane of the woman's existence by the modern-day leftist feminist. I admit that if a woman who works a full-time job gets pregnant, yes, she has to take maternity leave and will miss out on the meetings that took place during that time. But let's look at why maternity leave was created in the first place. It was created in order to protect women in the workplace, so that they can be a mom and return to their job. It was created so that they would get paid in full during their maternity leave. I fully support paid family leave and think that it is essential in order for women to work and also have children. If we did not give women maternity leave, we would be putting an undue burden on her, deterring women from having children and also working, creating a situation where women really wouldn't be able to do both. It is ironic how the leftist feminist takes a blessing like maternity leave and turns it into a curse.

So let's not pretend that maternity leave is ruining your life. It isn't. It's completely different to take a few months or even a year, off from the workplace than to take twenty years off from the workplace. Leftists often conflate the two, but the situations are not the same. I agree that if you haven't worked for twenty years, then it's going to be difficult to jump back in and catch up to your male counterparts who have been in the workforce that whole time. But if you take maternity leave or a year off, you can jump back in. I fully support whichever decision women make, whether that is to take a little time off and jump back into the workplace or a lot of time off, perhaps to be a stay-at-home mom. We should celebrate both, but the Left often ruthlessly beats up women who choose the latter or act as though women who chose the former are being held back by something great like maternity leave.

Or consider the teenage girl who is pregnant. I think of the movie *Juno*. The main character, a sixteen-year-old girl named Juno, considered getting an abortion, chose not to, and went to school while pregnant. She gave the child up for adoption and continued high school, dating a guy who was one of her closest friends. It was certainly an emotional and physical journey for her to have a baby, but it didn't preclude her from continuing her high school education.

Leftists who are pro-abortion promote the idea that motherhood is at best a drawback and at its worst a curse. And certainly they think this is true of motherhood when it is unplanned. They even think it warrants killing. Celebrating both men and women, as well as children, is important in order for our society to combat the toxic messaging of the far Left. We are often so consumed with discussing the war on women that we forget that there is a full-fledged war on babies.

CHAPTER TEN

MYTH: Abortion empowers women. Abortion is not something to be embarrassed about but celebrated as a reflection of our female strength and personal choices.

"Oh, it is excellent to have a giant's strength, but tyrannous to use it like a giant."[161]

—WILLIAM SHAKESPEARE, *Measure for Measure*

In the previous chapter we discussed arguments commonly made by the powerful left-wing feminists of the 1960s and 1970s. But today we hear a very aggressive, much more celebratory argument in favor of abortion from leftist feminists. This is the notion that abortion empowers women. Abortion is a form of strength, of female empowerment. It is an expression of women's control over themselves, over their bodies, and over their futures. Left-wing feminism embraces this ideology and the two are almost inseparable today. Abortion is something women should be proud of. Something not to feel bad about. Abortion is lauded as a form of power, and not exclusively women's power. They argue that abortion helps men, too, not just women. Men can be grateful to a woman they slept with who got an abortion.

We hear this a lot these days, especially from young women who see themselves as abortion activists. They're not just pro-choice; they're pro-abortion. They wear signs that say "abortion is freedom." We see this in the campaign called "Shout Your Abortion," which Oprah promoted in her magazine and on Oprah.com. The idea is that you should own your abortion. Work it. Make it part of your feminine strength.

Amelia Bonow, who founded the movement in 2015, wrote, "Plenty of people still believe on some level if you're a good woman, abortion is a choice that should be accompanied by some level of sadness, shame, or regret. But you know what? I have a good heart and having an abortion made me happy in a totally unqualified way."[162] Since then, Shout Your Abortion has grown into an organization that describes itself as "a movement working to normalize abortion through art, media, and community events all over the country."[163] The organization also sells merchandise, with award buttons like "I Had an Abortion and I'm Great" and foam fingers that point skyward and proclaim: "Thank God for Abortion."

The Shout Your Abortion website also has a slew of articles. Here's a list:

"2 abortions in 1 month and I'm fine!"
"I had an abortion and it wasn't scary, it was empowering"
"About to have a third abortion"
"I wouldn't change a thing"
"Having had an abortion I feel more connected to myself than ever before"

"My abortion made me love myself more"
"It doesn't really matter what your reason for having an
    abortion is"
"Live your truth"

There is also a movement called Thank God for Abortion.[164] This movement's Instagram frequently posts pictures of women holding babies, sometimes posing with crosses, halos, and other religious symbols resembling the Virgin Mary in order to appropriate these images, flout them, and say that God is for abortion.[165] *People* recently ran a piece titled "26 Celebrities Share Their Abortion Stories to Help End the Stigma."[166]

This movement seeks to normalize abortion, to make it seem as if it is nothing out of the ordinary in a woman's life experience, like it's not only morally okay but also something to be celebrated. This is the reality of what is going on in our country, and these are the voices our media outlets are amplifying. Outlets like this would never present views like mine, a pro-life position, in this kind of positive way or give me the megaphone that they have because what I am saying does not fit their agenda. Many good-hearted Democrats can't believe this is happening in our country, but it is. Abortion is now openly described as a positive good. It would be inaccurate to say that these voices are pro-choice. They are pro-abortion.

Recently, the actress Michelle Williams gave a speech at the Golden Globes while accepting an award for best actress in a series. She used the occasion to talk about her abortion and to celebrate her "choice." Williams said upon receiving her Golden Globes statue, "When you put this in someone's hands, you're acknowledging the choices that they make as an actor, moment by moment, scene by scene, day by day, but you're also acknowledging the choices they make as a person. . . . I wouldn't have been able to do this without employing a woman's right to choose."[167]

Leftists may wonder why conservatives find Hollywood satanic. It is primarily because of moments like this, where Michelle Williams appears to say essentially that she killed a child growing inside her in order to win a golden statue. She used her acceptance speech to position herself as an advocate for abortion and to encourage other women to do the same. She was seemingly proud of having had an abortion and in effect said that it enabled her career and her success, and of course, there she was holding the precious golden statue. What will little girls who saw her give that speech on TV, girls who hope to be an actress or win an award one day, think? "That's what I need to do to achieve my dreams."

Girls are bombarded with the messaging that abortion is empowering, spinning abortion as the road to the pinnacle of success. *Glamour* magazine wrote, "The internet exploded with praise for the moment—perhaps the most memorable of the night."[168] Actors, pundits, and leftist activists posted on social media about Michelle Williams's speech. Actress Reese Witherspoon wrote, "What a speech by #Michelle Williams! Thank you for being a champion of women, you are an inspiration."[169] Elizabeth Banks called Williams an "icon."[170] Golden Globes presenter Tiffany Haddish yelled, "Preach!" in the middle of Williams' speech.

Every little girl should know that she does not need to kill another person to be successful, beautiful, smart, or admirable. Or to win a golden statue.

A True Feminist

Let's look at this question of whether abortion really empowers women. We can begin by consulting the original feminists to see how they looked at the issue. Abortion is often portrayed as something that is a natural outgrowth of the women's rights movement, and yet we discover that all the original feminists, from Susan B. Anthony to Elizabeth Cady Stanton, were pro-life. They knew about abortion, rare as it was in those days, and were vehemently against it. Anthony and Stanton fought for women's economic opportunity and political opportunity. But they also knew that abortion was anti-woman and anti-life. Elizabeth Cady Stanton wrote, "It is degrading to women that we should treat our children as property to be disposed of as we fit" and referred to abortion as no different from "infanticide."[171] The newspaper that Anthony and Stanton ran together refused to run ads for abortifacients. Susan B. Anthony wrote in the newspaper *The Revolution* that abortion burdens the woman's "conscience in life, and soul in death."[172] And Sarah F. Norton, who worked with Susan B. Anthony on getting Cornell to admit women, took a similar position.[173]

Mary Wollstonecraft, who wrote *A Vindication of the Rights of Woman* and was perhaps the first feminist philosopher, also wrote disapprovingly of abortion. She said that women who "destroy the embryo in the womb or cast it off when born" lack strength and dignity. Elizabeth Blackwell, the first woman to receive a medical degree in the United States, wrote in her diary that she was filled with indignation over what she called "the gross perversion and destruction of motherhood by the abortionist."[174]

Stanford University scholar Michael McConnell writes in "How Not to Promote Serious Deliberation About Abortion" that "the nineteenth century anti-abortion movement was strongly supported by the women's movement."[175]

The original feminists realized that women's rights begin in the womb. As we see today with the radical pro-abortion leftists who call themselves "feminists," true feminism has been hijacked. I consider myself an original feminist in line with the desire for political and economic opportunity for women. But I cannot align myself with the radical leftist feminism that is fundamentally anti–human rights. We need to take back true feminism.

Abortion Is Power

We talk about empowerment a lot today, especially in the context of women's empowerment. It is brought up in the abortion debate as if abortion automatically equals empowerment or somehow produces empowerment. But what is empowerment, really? Simply, empowerment is based on the idea of power. Empowerment, as the word is used today, also has an inherent positive connotation. But we have to look at how power is used to see if true empowerment really applies here.

Let's say, for example, that you're standing at the edge of a precipice holding a baby, not an unborn baby but let's say a one-year-old, in your hands. You have the power to drop it over the cliff and send it plunging to its death. If you drop it, it will be gone. You clearly have immense power. That is without question. You're holding somebody else's whole life, their whole future, in your hands. But would you consider it a form of *empowerment* to let go, to exercise this power? This is nothing more than tyrannical power if used in this way. It is merciless killing. This is not empowerment.

"Oh, it is excellent to have a giant's strength," Shakespeare writes in *Measure for Measure*, "but tyrannous to use it like a giant."[176] We keep hearing from our culture that women should be empowered, and I agree. But is it empowerment to take innocent children's lives? Of course, as women we have power over them. They're largely helpless. But what if we use that power to kill them? What does that make us? Women do have the power to kill the innocent, but that doesn't make us powerful in the way we ought to be. We should seek the power to do good in the world and to improve the lives of others, not to take them.

I was pretty appalled when I saw that a woman named Emily Letts uploaded a video of her in-hospital abortion procedure. Emily is a twenty-five-year-old pro-abortion activist and works as a counselor at the Cherry Hill Women's Center in New Jersey. I was ready to watch the video, squinting so as to prepare myself for what I was about to see, but the video briefly showed her from the waist up in the operating room, and all that was shown was her smiling; the video then cut to her talking directly to the camera in a monologue fashion, so we didn't see the abortion take place. In her monologue she says that she did this "to show women that there is such a thing as a positive abortion story."

One might think that she got an abortion because she didn't see the baby as a life. But remarkably, she says in the video, "I feel in awe of the fact that I can make a baby. I can make a life." She adds, "I knew what I was going to do was right. Because it was right for me, and no one else."[177] She couldn't be more correct in saying that the decision was only right for her and no one else. Clearly what was "right" for the baby inside her did not affect her decision. She wanted to exercise her strength over the baby. And she did. It's dead.

Emily proceeded to take on a lot of media interviews including with HuffPost and *Cosmopolitan* magazine. She told *Cosmo*, "Every time I watch the video, I love it."[178] Was one negative word written about her by the mainstream media? Nope. She admitted that she was not on any form of birth control and that the man was never involved in her decision.[179]

After seeing her video and reading her interviews, all I could think of was Lady Macbeth, a character in one of Shakespeare's plays. Before she gets ready to participate with her husband in the murder of the king, she talks about suppressing her feelings and specifically about extinguishing her feminine instincts. She has to defeminize herself in a sense, producing a kind of extinction of nature in order to carry out this dastardly deed. For Lady Macbeth, femininity is sweet; it's empathetic. But for her to be able to carry out the awful deed, the awful murder, she finds that she must stamp out her femininity, developing a hardness if you will, that will enable her to kill. What does Lady Macbeth want? She wants power. She wants to have access to the throne. Shakespeare's account is a macabre demonstration of how killing can lead one to murder and destroy one's own nature.

After the murder, we see Lady Macbeth trying to wash her hands. "Out, damn'd spot," she shrieks.[180] There is no blood on her hands in the physical sense, but she thinks there is, and in her washing her hands she is trying to rid herself of the deed she's done. This is Lady Macbeth's attempt to stifle her own conscience, to forget the killing she did. And I think deep down this is what Emily Letts, the Shout Your Abortion movement, and the leftist feminist campaign to celebrate abortion are all about. They are about "out, damn'd spot." They're about celebrating something so awful in order to stifle one's own conscience. They're about extinguishing one's empathy and natural disposition of love and affection to your child so that one can become desensitized and, in celebrating it, not have to face the guilt.

When I think of ultimate power, omnipotence, if you will, and what that means, I think about God's power. Whether or not you believe in God, I am referring to the concept of ultimate power. One of God's powers is the power to create: God's creation not only of the universe and its complexities but also of life on Earth and specifically human life and each unique human life. This is a marvelous demonstration of divine power. Remarkably, it's a power that women, and only women, to some extent share. Women and only women have the power to physically give birth to life. Where would the world be without women? And so to take the power to bring life into this world and then use that power to kill that same life is a twisted evil. It is a true abuse of power. If women's empowerment is killing your baby in the modern American "feminist" movement, I want no part of it. It is not empowerment. When we become advocates for the taking of innocent lives, we cancel out any beauty or exquisiteness we once had in our feminine power, and it becomes black as soot.

The Patriarchy

Abortion, far from being "women's empowerment," actually supports the concept of the patriarchy. Leftist feminists argue that abortion is a way to "bring down the patriarchy," for women to not have to be controlled by men, and for the structure to be turned upside down. But the truth is abortion doesn't support women, and it ultimately supports a structure of male domination and male authority. And today's leftist feminists who promote abortion have acquiesced in this.

The hard truth is that men who can get away with cajoling or even coercing their partner to have an abortion are able to have sex without consequences. They don't have to deal with the child. They don't have to even pay child support. They don't have to be responsible to women. They don't have to be responsible for fatherhood. Think of the common sight of a couple in a bar. They flirt. One thing leads to another; they have sex in his or her apartment. The night ends. The woman discovers she's pregnant, shoot. She texts the man; she wants to talk. They meet after work, and he goes, "Hey, here's $500, go take care of it." This happens all too often.

Is this acceptable? Is this what feminists should fight for? For men to have sex with women and then treat them like mules for hire? Ultimately, to pay them off to "get rid of the contents of their womb"? The legal scholar Catharine MacKinnon says of *Roe v. Wade*, "*Roe* does not free women. It frees male sexual aggression. The availability of abortion removes the one remaining legitimate reason that women have had for refusing sex besides the headache."[181] What she's saying is that abortion encourages male irresponsibility, leaving women to get abortions, something they might not otherwise do, just because it is more convenient for men. I know that many men reading this can probably relate to this sentiment.

Think of all the men out there who are thankful for abortion—CEOs, movie executives, sexual predators like Harvey Weinstein. These are male jerks who like abortion because it enables their promiscuous lifestyle and lets them use women as playthings. Why should empowered women enable these people? Men who force abortion on women are the dregs of society. And ironically, feminists have become their enablers.[182] Notice that feminists who champion abortion rarely mention the fact that it was seven men who voted to legalize abortion. Seven men who probably knew that other men would benefit from it.

The worst men in society love abortion. There was a case in Indiana where a man killed his pregnant girlfriend and was sentenced to sixty-five years in prison. Why did he do it? Because she was past her sixth month and it was too late for her to get an abortion in her state.[183] He felt so entitled to be able to kill this child that he went ahead and killed them both. Abortion, and the feeling of entitlement to abortion, by men as well, has unleashed a culture of violence.[184]

I'm reminded of the novel *The Great Gatsby*, when Nick Carraway says, "They were careless people, Tom and Daisy. They smashed up things and creatures and then retreated back into their money or their vast carelessness, or whatever it was that kept them together and let other people clean up the mess they had made."[185] The fetus, the unborn that ends up in the dumpster, that's the mess that people make in our society today. These men who benefit from abortion are the moral successors to Tom and Daisy Buchanan.

"Abortion empowers women" is merely leftist media messaging. What we are getting is public propaganda that doesn't resemble the reality of the world. In a way, it reminds me of all the rhetoric we hear from some of the same people that prostitution is a form of empowerment. I ask myself—What is a more accurate picture of the prostitution community? Is it really women who are championing their freedom? Or is it women who are destitute, desperately in need of funds, feeling they have to do this in order to survive? This is not even the idea of having a lot of sex, it is the idea you have to have sex with whoever can shell out a few bucks. It doesn't matter how fat, ugly, and smelly the guy is. You gotta let him stick his penis inside you. Feminists call this "freedom." They call this "empowerment." Really? I would much rather empower these women to break free from the pimp that often controls a group of prostitutes, be rehabilitated and given nutrition they often lack, be able to go back to school, and have a life beyond prostitution.

The reality of abortion is similar. It's not an expression of freedom. It's not empowerment. It's a girl who is terrified going into an abortion clinic on a Saturday morning, who's going to have to lie on a stretcher, who's going to either have an invasive form of surgery or, if she goes in early enough, take an abortifacient pill only to go home and have a painful, bloody, flushing-out experience on her bathroom toilet, quietly moaning and weeping, hoping nobody hears her. That's what feminists today call empowerment. This is a sick, twisted lie that the pro-abortion movement is selling. This is not what the original feminists like Susan B. Anthony and Elizabeth Cady Stanton fought for.

Empowerment

Statistically, abortion does not empower women. Most babies aborted around the world are girls. Look at China, the most populous country in the world, where there is widespread killing of the unborn, mostly girls. But I am referring to more than China. In all countries where abortion is legal after the gender can be detected, there is the possibility of sex selection. "I want a boy. I don't want a girl." And this can be carried further to other kinds of selection. "I don't want a gay child. I don't want a disabled child. I want a designer baby." It is horrific that more black babies than white babies are aborted. What lie have the Democrats sold to women in order to bring this about? That it's about empowerment.

But is this really empowerment? No. This is eugenics. And this is reprehensible.

According to *Crisis Magazine*, Hillary Clinton invited Mother Teresa to have lunch with her at the White House while she was First Lady. Long before she ran for president herself, Hillary asked Mother Teresa why she thought there had not yet been a female president of the United States. The nun, of diminutive stature but more courageous than anyone, did not hesitate in her response and said, "Because she has probably been aborted."[186]

If we genuinely want to see women's empowerment, we need to put a stop to aborting baby girls who will be our future leaders. Truly strong women fight for the rights of the next generation of women.

If we are going to consider empowerment in a completely transparent way, most people would agree that empowerment is facing your situation and being stronger because of it. If you want to be a stronger person and really be empowered, take the high road and have your baby. You don't have to raise it, but if you can, do so. Many women can attest to the fact that motherhood has made them a stronger person, as it has presented challenges that they never would have faced otherwise, but it also presents them with empowering rewards and a remaking of their inner life that they never might have expected. Life is full of challenges, and it is how we meet them, respond, and rise to the occasion that defines us. When we choose to bestow death on another, it may feel powerful, but this feeling is empty and is not rooted in true empowerment that is life-giving to the soul.

In 2018, Kylie Jenner uploaded a YouTube video titled "To Our Daughter" that got eighty-nine million views. Kylie, the youngest of the infamous Kardashian siblings, got pregnant when she was twenty years old with the child of rapper Travis Scott. The video is beautifully done and is narrated by Kylie's friends and family speaking to Stormi, Kylie's daughter, almost as a love letter to her. We see Kylie go in for her ultrasound with her mom, and she hears the heartbeat. Her friend says, "When you're twenty years old, you're just figuring out your life. You don't know what you want. You're an indecisive teenager, you're just becoming a young adult. But there was one thing your mom knew for sure, and that was you."[187] The end of the video is when Kylie gives birth, and you can hear baby Stormi's cry and see her pudgy arm moving while in Kylie's arms.

I found the video to be a beautiful testament to the fact that Kylie chose life for her daughter. While we aren't all celebrities and Kylie isn't perfect, we can all look at the choice that Kylie made versus the choice to abort and see the beauty in it.[188] She told *Vogue Australia* in 2019, "I feel like having a daughter has made me love myself more....I want to be an example for her."[189] The pro-life author Randy Alcorn said, "Whenever I see an unmarried woman carrying a child, my first response is one of respect. I know she could have taken the quick fix without anyone knowing, but she chose to let an innocent child live."[190] I couldn't agree more.

I often think about women's empowerment, precisely because the Left uses this phrase so frequently to advocate for abortion. Though they are poisoning the term, we must take it back because true women's empowerment is so important. Many people say that women's empowerment means more women being in positions of power, and that is something we should strive for, but I also think it matters how we get there. We cannot justify killing others in order to get there, literally destroying babies' physical bodies and placing them at the altar of a fake version of empowerment.

THE CHOICE

I will be a successful woman, more successful than my great-grandmother would have ever dreamed, and I sure as heck will not kill my baby in the process. If the Left thinks that I need to do so, they are wrong. If killing my baby is what is required of me to be "empowered" in this day and age, then I want nothing to do with the word. Because taking innocent life is not empowerment. It's a charade. It's a farce. Seneca, the great philosopher, said, "All cruelty springs from weakness." This is true.

We gain power by being academically, politically, and economically successful. We also gain moral power by our strength of character. And one way we achieve that kind of power is to speak up and stand up for what is right. I have no doubt that we will face the cost of our decisions, when the radical Left beats up on us, denounces us, even tries to hinder us from success because of our pro-life views. But we can be empowered by knowing we're speaking up for those who have no voice, and we can be empowered by knowing that we are doing the right thing behind closed doors. The right thing is often the most difficult decision to make. It's clearly the harder path. But many times, in taking that path, we find ourselves becoming internally stronger. We find ourselves discovering true women's empowerment. From my own personal experience, I can say that defending the weak actually makes you strong. I am stronger than ever.

CHAPTER ELEVEN

MYTH: Planned Parenthood is not primarily an abortion organization; it is a women's health organization. Defunding Planned Parenthood would hurt minority communities, the people who benefit from it the most.

> "We don't want the word to get out that we want to exterminate the Negro population, and the minister is the man who can straighten out that idea if it ever occurs to any of their more rebellious members."
>
> —MARGARET SANGER, founder of Planned Parenthood[191]

If there is one organization above criticism for pro-choicers, it's Planned Parenthood. The organization pretends to be a health care operation, like the Red Cross. In reality, it is the biggest abortion mill in America. What is arguably worse is that its ancestry runs straight back to the most gruesome and violent racism in American history.

Pro-lifers understand this and view Planned Parenthood as the embodiment of modern evil. The satirical outlet *Babylon Bee* has joked that King Herod would receive Planned Parenthood's "lifetime achievement award."[192] King Herod is known for slaughtering innocent babies in the Bible, and the reason the grotesque comparison resonates is because Planned Parenthood is in the business of killing babies. Therefore, Planned Parenthood would look at King Herod as a role model.

Despite pro-life opposition, Planned Parenthood is the corporate giant of the abortion industry. It currently has over six hundred clinics all around the country.[193] To put that in perspective, Apple, which supplies many of us with smartphones and computers, has only 272 stores across the country. Planned Parenthood remains influential because it has huge megaphones at its disposal, primarily much of America's show-business empire, the glitzy arbiter of modern culture. The core of this support, of course, is Hollywood. Planned Parenthood recently launched a pro-abortion campaign collaborating with the designer Marc Jacobs and singer Miley Cyrus. Cyrus designed T-shirts and hoodies that say "DON'T F*CK WITH MY FREEDOM," picturing her topless and covering her breasts by holding grapefruit halves. One hundred percent of the profits from this vulgarity go to Planned Parenthood.[194]

In order to promote the upcoming collection, Cyrus posted a photo to her ninety-five million followers on Instagram, featuring herself seductively licking a cake. The icing on the cake says "Abortion Is Healthcare" with a caption reading, "Very special collab with @PlannedParenthood."[195] Cyrus told Jimmy Fallon on the *Tonight Show* that she's "a good face" for abortion and Planned Parenthood.[196]

Planned Parenthood also launched the #BansOffMyBody

campaign, which featured an open letter signed by 140 celebrities, including Ariana Grande, Lady Gaga, Nicki Minaj, Demi Lovato, Selena Gomez, Macklemore, and Billie Eilish, protesting the passage of state laws restricting abortion.[197] When Alabama recently voted to restrict abortion, Planned Parenthood and its celebrity entourage were outraged. Some celebrities boycotted working in the state, while others took the opportunity to raise money for Planned Parenthood. Singer Ariana Grande donated the proceeds from her Atlanta, Georgia, concert to Planned Parenthood, which amounted to about $250,000.[198]

Corporations have also been backing Planned Parenthood. The CEOs of over 180 companies, including Yelp, Warby Parker, Postmates, Glossier, Bloomberg L.P., Square Inc., and others, took out a full page ad in the *New York Times* calling for an end to bans on abortion.[199] And if you think celebrities and corporations love Planned Parenthood, look at Democratic politicians who love it even more. Senator Elizabeth Warren loves Planned Parenthood so much that she was excited to celebrate her birthday there.[200] Warren even says that if she ever becomes president, she'll wear a Planned Parenthood scarf for her inauguration.[201]

But how has Planned Parenthood achieved this totemic status? The answer is threefold. First, Planned Parenthood insists that abortion is not its main focus. Second, Planned Parenthood prides itself as a "women's health care organization." And third, Planned Parenthood claims that minorities are "most in need of its services" and, according to it benefit from its services the most.

We have all heard these claims, but are any of them true? The reality is that abortion is the lifeblood of Planned Parenthood, not its other services. Second, and shockingly, Planned Parenthood places little or no value on health care, not even the health of its female clients. Third, and worst of all, Planned Parenthood uses its power and influence to set up clinics in minority areas in order to target the abortion of black babies specifically.

"Abortion Is Not Planned Parenthood's Focus; Its Other Services Are."

How ironic that the one organization that is the single largest provider of abortions in the country, also fighting the hardest for abortion rights in politics, pretends not to be about abortion at all. That's the great hoax. It emphasizes its "other services" and claims that abortion is only 3 percent of what it does. This claim is very important to Planned Parenthood because it relates to its federal funding. According to the Hyde Amendment, abortions cannot be federally funded except in rare cases, so Planned Parenthood needs to emphasize its "other services" in order to keep getting federal funding. This false narrative has had huge payoff in taxpayer dollars. Between 2013 and 2015, Planned Parenthood raked in $1.3 billion for these "other services." While the funding is not to be used on abortions specifically, this obvious windfall from the government frees it up to use its other funding for abortions.

However, Planned Parenthood doesn't separate its abortion services from its other services, as it is required to do. Title X of the Family Planning Services and Population Research Act allocates funding for family planning services but specifies that those same services cannot refer patients for abortions. When the Trump administration ordered that Planned Parenthood separate its abortion activities from its family planning services if it wanted to continue to receive Title X funding, Planned Parenthood refused.

It really doesn't make sense for Planned Parenthood to refuse if it is true that its other services are what it cares about so much. Planned Parenthood chose to sacrifice about $60 million, which it was getting under Title X, in order to keep its other services comingled with abortion referrals. Title X is what Planned Parenthood calls "the gag rule" because it makes it feel like it's being gagged since abortion is so key to its services. No corporation would take a stance that threatens its core business. But abortion is Planned Parenthood's core business. If it were peripheral to the organization, it would separate the service or give it up. But it won't.

When Planned Parenthood's former president, Dr. Leana Wen, was asked about whether Planned Parenthood is focusing more on "other services," she told BuzzFeed News, "The last thing I want is people to get the impression that we are backing off of our core services. We will always be here to provide abortion access," adding, "It's who we are."[202]

Let's look at Planned Parenthood's famous claim that performing abortions is merely 3 percent of what it does. So, just how does Planned Parenthood arrive at this statistic? Planned Parenthood considers any discreet interaction with the clinic a "service." For example, if you go in for an abortion, it would likely give you a pregnancy test, an STD test, and a contraceptive device. If this happens, it would count the abortion performed as 25 percent of the services you received, counting each of those other items as a separate service. Planned Parenthood gives birth control out like candy, so every time it does that and a woman takes it, it's considered a "service." This kind of counting doesn't take into account the extensiveness of procedures, as getting a pregnancy test should hardly be considered a procedure equal to that of an abortion, considering you can get a pregnancy test at CVS for $10 and the most common abortion procedure is surgical.

Even the *Washington Post*, a pro-choice publication, gave Planned Parenthood's 3 percent figure three Pinocchio's, meaning that it found the figure to be "significant factual error" with "obvious contradictions."[203] The *Post* explains, "The 3 percent figure that Planned Parenthood uses is misleading in comparing abortion services to every other service it provides."

So, just how many babies does Planned Parenthood abort? According to numbers in its own 2018–2019 report, it performed 345,672 abortions that year.[204] In 2017–2018 it reported performing 332,757 abortions.[205] According to the Guttmacher Institute, there were 862,320 abortions performed in the United States in 2017.[206] Abortions in the United States are generally around 800,000 per year if we look at the last ten years.[207] This means that Planned Parenthood performs about 40–50 percent of all abortions in the United States, making it the single largest abortion provider.[208] There is no other chain of abortion clinics that comes close to matching Planned Parenthood in the number of abortions performed per year.

We can easily see what services Planned Parenthood focuses on by visiting its website. If Planned Parenthood is genuinely focused on broader "health care for women," then why is it that when you go to its website and click Get Care, the first option that comes up is "Abortion Clinics Near You"?[209] It does not say "Mammogram Near You" or "Pelvic Exam Near You." Aside from the fact that Planned Parenthood does not provide something as fundamental as mammograms, Planned Parenthood is clearly focusing on directing women to come to it specifically for abortions.[210]

Not only does Planned Parenthood encourage abortion on a grand scale, it routinely performs late-term abortions and is stepping up these numbers. A few years ago, Planned Parenthood had eighteen clinics that performed abortions after twenty weeks, and that number jumped to thirty-seven in 2018.[211] It also openly opposes any bans on late-term abortion to this day. They It believes that abortions should be performed to the moment of live birth.

Planned Parenthood used to support the killing of infants outside the womb, a horrific procedure. But, to its dismay, it became illegal in 2003, when President Bush signed into law a prohibition of killing babies outside the womb, such as in circumstances where the baby survived a botched abortion and the abortionist wasn't able to fully kill it in the womb. Undercover journalist David Daleidon recorded top Planned Parenthood executives on video bargaining over prices of fetal tissue from aborted baby parts. What we learn from this video is that Planned Parenthood is literally putting a price tag on fetal tissue taken from the remains of aborted babies in its clinics.[212] It is putting price tags on hearts and brains. One Planned Parenthood executive, when asked how much she wants for the fetal tissue, replies, "a Lamborghini."[213] Planned Parenthood has gone after Daleidon in various legal battles to cause him to go bankrupt because they're so angry that he exposed their top people on video.

In addition to performing late-term abortions, some Planned Parenthood staffers show a gruesome delight in their abortion work. Former Planned Parenthood director Abby Johnson has shared anecdotes of the kind of language employees used, such as referring to the freezer containing aborted baby parts as "the nursery." It's almost macabre to refer to the freezer with the dismembered parts as the nursery, as it shows the clear mental connection between abortion and killing babies. Abby Johnson also recalled a "supervisor joking about the babies that we aborted and things like, you know, the security code on our alarm was 2229 because that spelled out 'baby.' And they thought that was just hilarious."[214]

Planned Parenthood also celebrates abortionists themselves and their organizations, including a holiday to celebrate abortion and the people who perform them. Planned Parenthood posted an image on Twitter of a big pink heart that says "I Heart My Local Abortion Provider" with "Planned Parenthood" written underneath.[215] Planned Parenthood also posted an article leading up to this holiday describing its abortionists as "passionate, caring, skilled professionals."[216]

"Planned Parenthood Is a Women's Health Care Organization."

We've seen that abortion is the centerpiece of Planned Parenthood, but let's examine its second claim, which is that it is a health care organization that focuses on women.

Is health care its number one concern? If Planned Parenthood genuinely cared about health care, then it would have complied with health care regulations during the coronavirus disease pandemic. On March 18, 2020, the Centers for Medicare & Medicaid Services (CMS) announced that all elective surgeries, including medical and dental procedures, should be delayed during the 2019 novel coronavirus disease (COVID-19) outbreak.[217] Planned Parenthood refused to heed this warning and continued performing its elective services.

The Ohio attorney general, for example, mandated that all "non-essential or elective surgeries and procedures that utilize personal protective equipment" be stopped during the outbreak in an effort to make sure all masks and needed equipment go toward health care workers facing the coronavirus pandemic. The attorney general's office clarified that this included elective abortions that were not threatening to the mother's health. Planned Parenthood, however, ignored the order with an official statement: "Planned Parenthood's top priority is ensuring that every person can continue accessing essential health care, including abortion."[218]

Planned Parenthood clinics in Ohio continued to use medical equipment, including gloves and masks, as well as other vital supplies, in order to perform abortions. Planned Parenthood continued to perform abortions in Ohio that were not life-threatening to the mother but were purely elective. By continuing to perform its abortion services every day, it had multiple people congregating in their facilities, coming in and out every hour, while the entire state was in lockdown and ordered to shelter in place. The Ohio Department of Health director, Amy Acton, said, "As countless other clinics across the state comply with this health order and prioritize the lives of their fellow Ohioans, Planned Parenthood continues to put profit and abortion above the safety of our society's most vulnerable members—children and the elderly."[219]

We can also turn to Planned Parenthood's actions in Illinois. It determined that it would close eleven of seventeen clinics and cease certain operations, including cancer screenings, during the coronavirus pandemic in order to conserve resources. But it announced that it would continue to perform abortions. In other words, genuine health care it decided to stop, but in the case of voluntary "treatments" like abortions, it decided to continue.[220]

Unlike other hospitals and medical facilities, Planned Parenthood directly funds Democratic pro-choice candidates in political elections. This is not something St. Jude Children's hospital would do, for example. It's very unusual for a "health care" organization to do this. It even has an entire page on its website dedicated to bashing Donald Trump.[221] There is even a graphic on the page titled "Here is what Donald Trump controls" with arrows to "YOU." It has a list of the things Trump has done, which are meant to be insults, but they actually just draw attention to his accomplishments. For example, it lists, "Targeting Planned Parenthood." Planned Parenthood says, "Donald Trump is the first U.S. President to release a budget that singled out Planned Parenthood for 'defunding.'" It lists, "Packing courts with anti-abortion judges" and mentions Neil Gorsuch and Brett Kavanaugh as having records of opposing abortion. It condemns Trump for being the first president to speak at the March for Life.

But is it really active in elections, you might ask? I thought it only focused on health care! Planned Parenthood actually considers influencing politics to be one of its main goals. Former president Gloria Feldt started its political wing so that it can elect pro-choice candidates. Planned Parenthood is reported to be contributing a whopping $45 million into the 2020 election by funding pro-abortion candidates.

If there is any question about which side it supports politically, Planned Parenthood Action tweeted on March 15, 2019, "From now until November, this is the goal: we must defeat Donald Trump."[222] Jenny Lawson, the Planned Parenthood Votes executive director, told *CBS News*, "The Trump administration has managed to undo so much over the last three years. The stakes have never been higher."[223]

The Federal Elections Commission (FEC) reported that zero percent of Planned Parenthood donations go to Republican candidates.[224] It is functioning as an arm of the Democrats. Cecile Richards, who was president of Planned Parenthood for twelve years, had clear political goals for the organization. After serving as president of Planned Parenthood she left to fund Supermajority, a political action group, and before becoming president of Planned Parenthood she worked for Democratic congresswoman Nancy Pelosi. Planned Parenthood even received grants from the Obama administration to promote Obamacare.

Not only does it fund pro-abortion Democratic candidates, but it also funds the fight against pro-life judges and cases related to abortion. It wants to influence the courts in its favor, so it does everything it can to funnel money in ways that are beneficial to its pro-abortion cause. This is not a secret. An entire section of its annual report is devoted to what it calls "advocacy." It claims *Roe* is at risk and that fighting back in courts is what is necessary. It is proud to report that it had over one thousand people standing outside the Judiciary Committee hearings to protest Kavanaugh's confirmation every day. It also organized marches throughout seventy-five communities across the country to protest his confirmation.[225] According to its own report, it has 140,357 "defenders signed up to take action at a moment's notice following a text from us." It has over 120 chapters at college campuses in order to get young people involved in elections, teaching them "deep organizing skills."[226] We can see that Planned Parenthood is a political arm of the pro-abortion Left. Does this sound like a "health care" organization to you?

On July 16, 2019, Planned Parenthood came out directly criticizing me and women who support President Trump, tweeting, '"Women for Trump' launched today, and the hypocrisy is stunning. Since taking office, the Trump admin has systematically taken away our health and rights—policies that hurt all women, including his own supporters."[227] As the youngest woman on the Advisory Board of Women for Trump, who deeply cares about women's empowerment, I find Planned Parenthood's view that in order to be an intelligent woman, you have to support the killing of innocent babies, flat-out ridiculous. There is nothing hypocritical about women opposing killing babies because killing babies is not synonymous with women's health, well-being, or our nature. We are nurturers, communicators, fighters, and preservers of life, not killers. The proclamation that all women must join in the fight to take innocent babies' lives degrades us all as women and is a proclamation we should all oppose.

Women have brains, just like men do, and can reason out the fact that Planned Parenthood is the largest abortion provider and does not stand up for women seeking aid or vulnerable infants in the womb. Women's rights extend to the little girl babies in the womb. Women deserve to be treated with dignity and given better options than abortion. President Trump protects life and supports women through policies he's passed like paid family leave, allowing working women to spend more time with their babies while still making money. But what about Planned Parenthood, you may wonder—does it value women?

Keeping Women Uninformed

If Planned Parenthood cared about the health and well-being of women, why would it vehemently oppose laws requiring doctors to show a woman her ultrasound? Why do it want to pull the wool over women's eyes? Many women do not know that the fetus in the womb has developed much at all because abortion clinics tell them otherwise. If this is truly a health care procedure and not a sting operation intended to mislead women, then women should be informed, as they would be about any other health care procedure, and not left in the dark.

This is why Republicans are advocating that women be shown an ultrasound before getting an abortion. The woman can still proceed with her abortion if she wishes. Kentucky passed this law and Democrats challenged it, but it was upheld in the Sixth U.S. Circuit Court of Appeals. Judge John K. Bush wrote that this law "requires the disclosure of truthful, non-misleading and relevant information about an abortion."[228]

Planned Parenthood says that showing women their ultrasound is "cruel." Why? It knows what the woman will see in that ultrasound: a baby. A woman seeing that, and in light of that, often changes her mind and walks out of the clinic. This is detrimental to Planned Parenthood's revenue and reputation, as well as the entire pro-choice ideology, so Democrats try to strike down these laws whenever they can.[229]

Planned Parenthood also opposes any laws requiring a waiting period to get an abortion. These laws are intended to ensure that the woman really wants to get one, is not being coerced, and has had time to think it over. This waiting period is typically twenty-four hours between the initial session and the abortion itself. Not a lot of time. Planned Parenthood opposes even this short window because it knows that if a woman goes home to think about what abortion is, even without having seen her ultrasound, she will likely not return the next day. This is why Planned Parenthood does not want to give you that chance to think it over. This is merely another attempt to manipulate women and coerce them into the operating room. Planned Parenthood has to think about its bottom line. More abortions, more money.

Planned Parenthood does not value the health and well-being of young women either. For example, the organization opposes laws requiring parental notification before an abortion is performed on a minor. Though abortion on a fifteen-year-old or younger is rare, Planned Parenthood still performs abortions on demand for minors, who do not have the right to vote or buy a beer but can undergo a surgical procedure without their parents knowing. This could be a scarring experience for a minor and have lifelong consequences for her. It also raises the question of whether this minor fully understands the procedure about to take place. Serious health complications could arise as well. What if the minor does not disclose or does not know her full health history and the procedure is performed at risk to her health? What if she is allergic to the type of anesthetic used? Parents have the right to know about other operations performed on their underage child, so why is abortion the exception?

Lila Rose, now the president of Live Action, exposed the hypocrisy of Planned Parenthood in a series of undercover videos, in which she showed how it treats women in cases of sexual abuse. Lila walked into a Planned Parenthood clinic and said that she needed an abortion because she was a fifteen-year-old girl having sex with a twenty-three-year-old boyfriend, making her a victim of statutory rape. Instead of referring her to where she might be able to get help or reporting the stated abuse, Planned Parenthood officials told her to lie about her age on the paperwork at the clinic so they could act like they had never heard anything about it and could move on with the abortion. This is what Planned Parenthood means when it says that it does "nonjudgmental care." Its nonjudgment extends even to protecting rapists.

You may wonder—But isn't Planned Parenthood required to meet the health care needs of women? If Planned Parenthood wasn't around, where would women go for health care? First, community health centers outnumber Planned Parenthood locations ten to one.[230] Second, if Planned Parenthood was necessary in order to serve the health care needs of women, how do some states with very few or no Planned Parenthood locations at all—North Dakota, Kentucky, South Carolina, and Kansas—manage without it?[231] The women in those states are getting their health care needs met. New York and California have the most Planned Parenthoods. Are women in California and New York getting better tested for cancer then? No, but they are having more abortions.

Planned Parenthood also supports the horrible practice of sex-selective abortions. In other words, a woman can choose to stay pregnant until she can find out the sex of the baby, and if it isn't the gender she wants, then she can abort it. In March 2016, the Indiana legislature passed a law by wide margins called the Sex-Selective and Disability Abortion Ban, preventing a woman from having a sex-selective abortion. Planned Parenthood promptly filed a lawsuit opposing this law as unconstitutional.[232]

Why would it do this? Shouldn't we all agree that targeting a baby girl because of her gender is discrimination? But Planned Parenthood stopped the law from going into effect. It then was tried in several courts and made it all the way to the Supreme Court. It was put on hold, and the court will certainly return to it soon. The sad reality is that in the world today, the majority of abortions are performed on baby girls, solely because of their sex. If we look at the effects of China's one-child policy, for example, we see generations without girls, a missing 160 million women, about the size of the female population in the United States.[233]

In America, no one should be discriminated against solely because of gender, according to the equal protection clause of the Fourteenth Amendment. I know that Planned Parenthood and other pro-choicers would argue that rights don't apply to a little girl in the womb because she is not a "person." But to that I say— she obviously has private parts and genitalia; she is in every way a girl and purely because of that is being targeted and killed based on her sex. Shouldn't we all oppose this brutal killing rooted in discrimination? If Planned Parenthood is genuinely for "women's rights," it would oppose sex-selective abortion, but instead its actions are quite the contrary as it is the biggest advocate for it, advocating for it all the way to the Supreme Court.

"Planned Parenthood Cares about Minority Communities. The Services It Provides Benefit Them the Most."

Last, Planned Parenthood claims to serve minority communities, even claiming that taking away its services would harm blacks the most. It features black women in its pamphlets and on its website and attempts to appeal to black women directly. Planned Parenthood is currently selling merchandise including T-shirts, water bottles, purses, and other items that are black or purple with the capitalized slogan "STAND WITH BLACK WOMEN."[234] It clearly thinks that abortion services are for black women. What does Planned Parenthood mean when it says this?

We can answer this question by looking to Planned Parenthood's founder, Margaret Sanger, who was proudly and unabashedly motivated by an ideology called eugenics. In her 1932 speech

"My Way to Peace," she lays out her eugenics creed as the way to achieve "world peace," which involves segregation and sterilization. She calls this controlling "the input and output of morons."[235] She wanted to create what she thought was a "perfect society." She wanted to create a society of the "fit," which she defined as rich, white, educated elites. Meanwhile the "unfit" must be stopped from ruining the rest of society.

In her 1922 book *The Pivot of Civilization*, Sanger wrote, "A lack of balance between the birth rate of the 'unfit' and 'fit' is admittedly the greatest present menace to the civilization."[236] She described the supposed problem of the "feeble-minded" on the one side producing too much and the "educated and well-to-do classes" reproducing less, resulting in a society that would have far more feeble-minded people than well-to-do people. She said that chaos would ensue "unless the feeble-minded are prevented from reproducing their kind."[237]

Margaret Sanger was obsessed with eugenics, as the titles of several of her articles show: "Some Moral Aspects of Eugenics" (June 1920), "The Eugenic Conscience" (February 1921), "The Purpose of Eugenics" (December 1924), "Birth Control and Positive Eugenics" (July 1925), and "Birth Control: The True Eugenics" (August 1928), to name a few.

She thought of blacks as the lowest of the low. Once Sanger realized she could not forcibly sterilize everyone she viewed as a human weed, she knew she had to convince blacks to sterilize themselves so that they would not procreate anymore and eventually die out. Sanger instigated what she termed "The Negro Project" in 1939, a project that merged with the efforts of Birth Control Federation of America. The goal was to limit the number of black babies born by making sure black women started using birth control. With the cooperation of the New York Urban League, Sanger set up one of her first birth control clinics in Harlem, New York, to target blacks.[238] After focusing on blacks in urban areas, she moved to blacks in rural areas.

Sanger co-drafted a report titled *Birth Control and the Negro* in which she stated, "Negroes present the great problem of the South," as they are the group with "the greatest economic, health, and social problems." She claimed that their population must be curtailed because they are largely illiterate and "still breed carelessly and disastrously."[239]

Sanger had nothing but positive recollections of her visit to the women of the Ku Klux Klan in Silver Lake, New Jersey, in 1926.[240] She said of the visit in her 1938 autobiography, "I believe I had accomplished my purpose. A dozen invitations to speak to similar groups were proffered."[241] She was right at home with them. Sanger did not write of any regrets of having spoken to them or any disagreements she had with them either. Their goals were the same as hers.

Sanger's overarching goal was to "exterminate the Negro population," as she wrote in a private letter to Clarence Gamble in 1939. She says that the nature of her organization is to target the African American community, writing, "The most successful educational approach to the Negro is through religious appeal. We don't want the word to get out that we want to exterminate the Negro population, and the minister is just the man who can straighten out that idea if it ever occurs to any of their more rebellious members."[242] Sanger convinced prominent blacks like W. E. B. Du Bois, Mary McLeod Bethune, and Reverend Adam Clayton Powell Jr. to spread her message of population control for blacks.

One might say that Planned Parenthood has changed and

isn't racist anymore. But sadly, Planned Parenthood is just as racist today as its founder was then. Eugenicists after World War II did not disappear but simply moved into the population control movement. World War II brought the informal referendum on racism to the forefront, and the public did not like what it saw. The civil rights movement of the 1960s solidified this, and racism was not acceptable in the public square by the 1970s and 1980s. As a result, the eugenics movement needed a different name, another justification for the same ideology of limiting population but with the same end goal. "Population control" became an acceptable way to argue that we need fewer people in the world without having to say the word "eugenics." Once the population control movement collapsed, the same people pivoted into the abortion movement as we know it today.

A key pivoter includes Planned Parenthood itself, which began by promoting eugenics and sterilization, then population control, and then abortion. Planned Parenthood follows this line of thinking in its history. Planned Parenthood's website under "Our History" confirms this. The American Birth Control League, which it describes as "an ambitious new organization that examined the global impact of population growth," and Margaret Sanger's Birth Control Research Bureau "merged to become Planned Parenthood Federation of America."[243] The same ideology of eugenics and extermination continued, but using a different strategy.

We can see the same act of pivoting regarding other prominent eugenics organizations. The American Eugenics Society, for example, changed the name of its scholarly publication from *Eugenics Quarterly* to *Social Biology*.[244] The journal's editor explained that eugenics goals could be achieved through different tactics.

Alan Guttmacher carried on the legacy of Margaret Sanger. He was vice president of the American Eugenics Society of which Margaret Sanger was a member. He became one of Planned Parenthood's most influential presidents, serving as president through the *Roe v. Wade* Supreme Court decision until 1974. He explicitly endorsed abortion for eugenic reasons.[245] Regarding abortion, he claimed that "the quality of parents must be taken into account," including "feeble-mindedness."[246] He claimed that the question of whether to allow abortion must be "separated from emotional, moral, and religious concepts."[247] He was purely focused on the social outcome.

But is the ghost of Margaret Sanger still alive today? Oh, yes it is. Let's look at where Planned Parenthood clinics are located today. Over 70 percent of Planned Parenthood locations are located in predominantly minority communities. Abortion is the leading cause of death for black Americans.[248] In New York City, more black babies are aborted than are born.[249] In some areas, a black baby is eight times more likely to be aborted than a white baby. This is not health care, this is Planned Parenthood purposefully putting its locations in predominantly black neighborhoods, targeting them, and succeeding. Margaret Sanger could never have dreamed that her organization would be this effective in exterminating the next generation of blacks. If Margaret Sanger were alive today, she would be happy to see that clinics today are exactly where she wanted them.

Planned Parenthood pretends it does this because it wants to "serve black women." But you don't help a community by killing its next generation. Alveda King, civil rights activist and niece of Reverend Martin Luther King Jr., explains that the leading cause of death for the black community isn't gang violence, gun violence, heart attack, stroke, diabetes, or HIV but abortion alone. About a third of abortions in America since *Roe v. Wade* have been on black babies, when blacks are 13 percent of the population.[250] These numbers are wildly disproportionate. King said, "The great irony... is that abortion has done what the Klan only dreamed of."[251]

King dispels the notion that blacks are more prone to wanting abortions, saying, "Now does it mean that African Americans are more immoral or don't care? Absolutely not. We are just regular, everyday people like everyone else. But Planned Parenthood moved into our community with the abortion killing centers and said, 'We're here to help you. Let's kill your baby, so you can have a better life.'"[252]

We all know that Planned Parenthood targets minority communities for a reason, and it's eugenics. Secretary of Urban Development Ben Carson told Neil Cavuto on Fox News, "One of the reasons that you find most of their clinics in black neighborhoods is so that you can find a way to control that population."[253] Benjamin Watson, a tight end for the Baltimore Ravens, spoke at the annual March for Life in Washington, DC, saying, "I do know that blacks kind of represent a large portion of the abortions, and I do know that honestly the whole idea with Planned Parenthood and Sanger in the past was to exterminate blacks," Watson said. "And it's kind of ironic that it's working."[254]

Supreme Court Justice Clarence Thomas wrote in his opinion of *Box v. Planned Parenthood* that "the use of abortion to achieve eugenic goals is not merely hypothetical. The foundations for legalizing abortion in America were laid during the early 20th-century birth-control movement.... Planned Parenthood founder Margaret Sanger recognized the eugenic potential of her cause."[255]

The proof that Planned Parenthood continues in the Margaret Sanger tradition is that it celebrates her still. Planned Parenthood's presidents including Gloria Feldt and Faye Wattleton share Sanger's ideology. Wattleton has claimed that she was "proud" to be "walking in the footsteps of Margaret Sanger."[256] Feldt has stated: "I stand by Margaret Sanger's side," leading "the organization that carries on Sanger's legacy."[257] Planned Parenthood's current president, Alexis McGill Johnson, even wrote an article in 2019 titled "In Defense of Margaret Sanger on Eugenics."[258] Planned Parenthood proudly carries the torch of Margaret Sanger.

In 1966, Planned Parenthood began presenting the Margaret Sanger Award annually to recognize, in its words, "individuals of distinction in recognition of excellence and leadership in furthering reproductive health and reproductive rights." It venerated Margaret Sanger in the 1960s, and clearly it venerates Margaret Sanger to this day. Not surprisingly, one of the recipients of the Margaret Sanger Award, the "highest honor," was Hillary Clinton. In her acceptance speech in 2009, Hillary Clinton said, "I admire Margaret Sanger enormously, her courage, her tenacity, her vision....I am really in awe of her."[259] Nancy Pelosi glowingly accepted the award in 2014. President Obama spoke to Planned Parenthood in 2013 and hailed the organization, commending its "extraordinary" and "remarkable work," saying it does a "great, great job."[260]

CHAPTER TWELVE

MYTH: The pro-life argument is inherently a religious one, and the only people who are pro-life are religious. Keeping abortion legal affirms the separation of church and state.

"As an atheist, I believe that we don't have the consolation of an afterlife. We have only one life to live. So it had better be good."[261]

—CHRISTOPHER HITCHENS, atheist and writer, *Crisis Magazine*

Some pro-choice advocates seek to dismiss pro-life arguments on the ground that the pro-life argument is based solely on religious grounds. They say pro-lifers are getting it from the Bible or some other religious tract and to impose that argument on the public violates the norms of democracy and specifically violates the doctrine of separation of church and state. Liz Hayes, who writes for a group called Americans United, puts it this way: "The aggressive abortion ban bills being considered in states across the country may not explicitly mention religion, but it's clear that these bills and the restrictive policies they propose are religiously motivated."[262] Americans United says on their website that they "use high-impact litigation, powerful lobbying, and grassroots advocacy to ensure that religion does not affect public policy."[263]

What Americans United may have going for them is that when you go to a pro-life demonstration or rally, you do see religious people there. You see nuns, you see people with rosaries, you see evangelical Christians praying to end abortion. If you listen to pro-life speeches, you will hear references to God. Clearly, there is a religious aspect to this debate. The Catholic Church has consistently opposed abortion throughout its history. Strong evangelical churches are also passionately against abortion. Orthodox Jews are a strong part of the pro-life cause. So there *is* a religious pro-life coalition. Many pro-lifers are held together by a philosophical worldview.

But this is equally true of the pro-choice camp. What we must realize is that no one can escape having a world-view. Even if you say you are unbiased, there is no such thing. You may say, well, "I'm not religious, Danielle," but even so, secularism is a worldview. Atheism is a worldview. Agnosticism is a worldview. A worldview is simply the larger way in which we view the cosmos, our purpose, and our life on Earth. People live based on their worldview and vote based on their worldview all the time, even if they don't realize it. When someone who is secular and pro-choice points the finger at a religious, pro-life person, they are naming themselves as Hypocrite of the Year because their political beliefs clearly stem from their religion, too, or hatred of it. They are not an unbiased observer, as much as they say they are. No one is.

Separation of church and state was created to protect religious freedom, not stamp it out. The term "separation of church and state" does not appear in the Constitution but is a phrase lifted from one of Jefferson's letters. The Constitution uses the phrase "no establishment," which is what we call the "no-establishment clause." So, what is it? It is the clause that says that the government cannot "establish" a national religion. This was put in place to protect religious freedom. For example, the Anglican Church in England, which is England's official religion, has state preference. Unlike England, the Founders intended for there to be no official religion in America. The Left has taken this to mean that secularism is the "religion of the state," but what the Founders intended was for people to be able to freely express their own religion, any religion or no religion at all. As Ronald Reagan said, "The Constitution was never meant to prevent people from praying. Its declared purpose was to protect their freedom to pray."[264]

We All Have a Conscience

I want to take a step back from religion specifically and think about morality. We must also remember that there is a sense of morality in each of us that precedes a belief in a religion. When we think about morality, we can think of the morality that comes from revelation or sacred scripture, or you might say from "on High"; and then there is the morality that comes to us from conscience, one might say "the little voice in your head." The morality that comes to us from conscience is innate to every human being. If human beings don't have conscience, they are considered sociopaths or psychopaths; in fact, in legal terms, we don't even hold them accountable for their behavior because to some degree, we don't even consider them to be able to know the difference between right and wrong as other humans do. Most of us don't fall into this category. Morality and conscience are part of the human experience, innately, whether or not we choose to be religious. We all have that little voice in our head telling us not to do something bad. This doesn't mean we listen to it; we may ignore it, even contort it, but the voice is somewhere in there.

Let's think about the Ten Commandments. While the commandments are a product of revelation, in that God revealed them to us through Moses, we also know these things to be true anyway. The first few commandments clearly deal with revelation and with God explicitly, but the later commandments—thou shalt not kill, thou shalt not commit adultery, though shalt not steal—are accessible to conscience. Personally, I didn't even learn them from the Bible. It wasn't that I read the Bible and then thought, "Wow, stealing is wrong. Wow, adultery is wrong. Wow, killing is wrong. I will try to follow this." I already knew those things through my own conscience. When we see them in the Ten Commandments, this in a sense confirms what we already hear from the voice in our head and reminds us to listen to that voice, giving us a more powerful reason to listen to it. I bring this up because sometimes in an effort to prevent theology from entering politics, what lobbyists are actually trying to do is stamp out morality altogether.

I am not saying that you have to agree with the content of the commandments or that you have to follow them, but we all can accept that we can talk about them. They can be part of moral debate and part of democratic discourse, just as any other person's moral arguments can. In fact, this is what democratic discourse is largely about: separating what's right from what's wrong and trying to build a structure of laws that reflects truth and goodness. This is different from forcing theology on someone, as no theology is forced upon anyone in America by the government—I am referring to pure discussion in the public square and the freedom of individuals to vote based on their conscience. How does expressing your conscience violate separation of church and state? Answer: it doesn't.

A Judeo-Christian worldview tells us so much about the dignity of every person, every child, created by God. But even if you do not believe in God, you can begin with your intuition that harming others or killing them is wrong. You see someone kicking a dog, you recoil. Beating an old lady over the head with a stick, you know that's wrong. You know this naturally, in a sense, without even having to think about it. Let's say you see a man with a knife stabbing a pregnant woman in the belly. You know that this is something more than stabbing her in the back or on the thigh.

Our laws acknowledge this. We've had laws across this country that basically say that if you kill a woman and her unborn child, it's a double homicide. Recently, New York changed its law on this score, but not because it had any different view of what was going on in the murder but rather because the New York legislature realized that having these laws on the books creates a contradiction with abortion. How can you treat it as a double homicide if the laws of New York don't acknowledge that the fetus is, in fact, a human person? And so New York had to change the law to make it compatible with its pro-abortion ideology.

Christopher Hitchens

I had the pleasure of getting know the famous atheist and prominent writer Christopher Hitchens because my dad and Hitchens would frequently debate each other in a series of apologetics debates on the existence of God. Hitchens passed away in 2011.

He wrote an article in *Crisis Magazine* called "A Left-Wing Atheist's Case against Abortion." Hitchens was an atheist and a materialist. By materialist he meant that he believed the material body is all there is, that even as human beings we don't really have a spiritual dimension. We are merely matter in the universe—and precisely because of that, we have to give human life, including developing human life, protection. Remarkably, Hitchens wrote, "As a materialist I hold that we don't have bodies, we *are* bodies. And as an atheist, I believe that we don't have the consolation of an afterlife. We have only one life to live. So it had better be good....If the unborn is a candidate member of the next generation, it means that it is society's responsibility."[265]

If we truly have only one life to live, and that is this life on Earth, to stamp out someone's existence is to commit the ultimate crime. If we are truly only bodies and without a soul, then every child that has been killed has not gone on to Heaven but only to the grave. Those who do not believe in an afterlife would call this "pure annihilation." It literally is, in every sense, the end. And this is irrevocable not only for the physical signs of life—your pulse, your brain waves—but also your conscience, thoughts, experiences, and future; it ends your whole life story. That is an incredibly depressing thought, and Hitchens rightly states that taking away someone else's existence, without cause, is unacceptable.

You may wonder, but why does Hitchens think the fetus is a person? Why does he concede this? Hitchens answers bluntly, "I think that at this point we know where babies come from." Honesty at its finest. Hitchens also discusses the fact that so many pro-choice advocates argue that the fetus behaves in ways that are inhuman, drawing attention to how it doesn't have the same complex thoughts as we do. Hitchens says to this, "Dialectics will tell you that you can't be meaningfully inhuman unless you are also potentially human as well. It's pointless to describe a rat or a snake, say, as behaving in an inhuman fashion." We don't argue about whether rats are human because they obviously are not. Every time we argue about whether a human is "really human," they always are.

When asked whether he would like to see *Roe v. Wade* overturned and returned to the states, he said, "I would prefer to see abortion as a federal issue. Nothing is more horrible than inconsistency on the life question." Hitchens says there should be a federal prohibition of abortion with the life of the mother, rape, and incest exceptions. "Now I know most women don't like having to justify their circumstances to someone. 'How dare you presume to subject me to this?' some will say. But, sorry, lady, this is an extremely grave social issue....There is a debased compassion at work. It tends to be one sided, exclusively focused on the female condemned, as they say, to domestic serfdom."

I completely agree with Hitchens on the fact that there must be a federal ban on abortion. We need *Roe v. Wade* overturned as well as a federal ban on abortion in the form of an amendment to the Constitution. Just as the Thirteenth Amendment ended slavery, the Fourteenth Amendment gave equal rights, the Fifteenth Amendment gave blacks the right to vote, and the Nineteenth Amendment gave women the right to vote, we need an amendment that protects the rights of the unborn. A child in the womb must be protected from intentional killing and violence. If the fetus truly is a person in the meaningful sense of the word, no state should be allowed to invalidate its personhood and take its life. The idea of abortion as a state's issue does not line up with the nature of the fetus, which is the fact that it has universal human dignity, just as you or I do. I recognize that *Roe v. Wade* must be overturned first, and the issue will then be a state's issue, and that will be the first victory. But we must not stop there. A federal ban is needed in order to protect the unborn.

Abortion is a human rights issue. It is a universal issue that we can all get behind. Everyone can be pro-life because of what we see, because of scientific and medical facts, because of observation, because of conscience, and because of empathy.

Christians in the Forefront

Religious people through our history have been at the forefront of great reform movements protecting life and protecting human rights in various forms. Churches, for example, were in the forefront of the abolition movement. If it hadn't been for the Christian abolitionists, we might still have slavery in this country. This is also true of civil rights. If it hadn't been for the churches, we might still have segregation and state-sponsored discrimination. So, the same people who fault the pro-life movement for invoking religion don't seem to be complaining about Reverend Martin Luther King Jr. for giving passionate sermons and invoking God in his struggle. I don't see them faulting abolitionist preachers for their activism on behalf of abolitionism. Christians lead the charge on many moral causes in American politics, and fighting moral wrongs is not easy.

Christians often lead the charge in fighting moral injustice around the world as well. Dietrich Bonhoeffer, the famous Nazi dissident and pastor, said, "Silence in the face of evil is evil itself." Desmond Tutu, the cleric and theologian, led an anti-apartheid movement in South Africa. The Christian politician and activist William Wilberforce led the anti-slavery movement in England. He said, "You may choose to look the other way but you can never say again that you did not know." We refuse to look the other way.

It sometimes takes deep conviction to push forward on these issues, a conviction drawn, you might say, not just from the world but in some cases from out of this world. It is the innermost churning of the soul and righteous indignation that are often needed to fight such a large injustice. Without that strength of spirit and conviction of what is right and wrong, it is difficult to make change.

Christians typically lead the charge, and then others get on board. I suspect that later on in history, those who did nothing for the pro-life movement, while we struggled and toiled, will try to take credit for what we have done for the unborn. Later on in history, everyone will want to identify with "the right side of history." We are on it now, when it's not accepted in the culture, when we are spat on and largely painted to be fanatics who want to hurt women. This could not be further from the truth, as so many pro-life advocates love women and children and are women themselves. But if others try to take the credit later, that only means we've succeeded in exposing abortion as a moral evil and have genuinely changed the culture. Father Frank Pavone, active in the pro-life movement, says, "It's time to change the fear of preaching about abortion into a fear of what will happen if we don't."

Billy Graham was asked to be a spiritual advisor to President Obama but found that he could not endorse Obama because of the former president's pro-abortion position; nevertheless, he said that he would like to pray with him. Billy Graham's son Franklin told the Associated Press that the Bible clearly teaches the value of human life. He said, "President Obama heard our position," and I told him, "It's a moral issue that we just can't back down on."

Referring to Obama's position on abortion, Graham said, "Those positions that he holds that are contrary to Biblical teaching, I hope that God will change his heart."[266]

Pope Benedict XVI said, "God's love does not distinguish between the infant in the mother's womb or the child or the youth or the adult or the older person. In each one God sees His image and likeness. Human life is a manifestation of God and His glory." Pope John Paul II said, "Give us the grace, when the sacredness of life is attacked, to stand up and proclaim that no one ever has the authority to destroy unborn life." Pope Francis says this of abortion: "Defend the unborn against abortion even if they persecute you, calumniate you, set traps for you, take you to court or kill you." A liberal himself in many ways, Pope Francis says, "It is not progressive to try to resolve problems by eliminating human life."

As a Christian, I am reminded of the fact that one unplanned pregnancy saved mankind. This was the birth of Jesus Christ. The miracle child, born unto a virgin. I am sure she was in shock at her pregnancy, and Joseph could have walked away. But we see the beautiful picture of the holy family. They are not in a palace or in a castle but in a barn. And unto us a king is born. The birth of Jesus is the most famous unplanned pregnancy, at least unplanned in the eyes of Mary and Joseph, and this unplanned pregnancy has been uplifted by millions for centuries. We see the uplifting not just of the child but of the mother as well. And when Jesus walks the Earth he loves every person, whether that is his mother, Mary, or the woman at the well who had five husbands.

When I think of the abortion issue and the helpless child, I think of Proverbs 30:8, "Speak up for those who cannot speak for themselves." A child is not a mistake, burden, nuisance, or punishment.

A child is a gift from God. If you find that you are fearing the opinions of men or fear that we will never win this battle and overturn *Roe v. Wade*, remember that there is a higher court than the Supreme Court, one that is ruled by the Lord.

The poet Dante writes that "the darkest places in Hell are reserved for those who maintain their neutrality in times of moral crisis." While the *Divine Comedy* is a poem, I think he speaks some truth in saying this. When you have the ability to help someone at no cost to yourself—in this case, cast a vote in favor of saving innocent babies from being killed—and choose not to, you actively forsake them.

THE LESSER OF TWO EVILS

"It is in the nature of the human being to seek a justification for his actions."

—ALEKSANDR SOLZHENITSYN, *The Gulag Archipelago*[267]

CHAPTER THIRTEEN

MYTH: I'm personally opposed to abortion, but I don't have the right to force my beliefs on someone else.

> "He who passively accepts evil is as much involved in it as he who helps perpetrate it. He who accepts evil without protesting it is really cooperating with it."[268]
>
> –Reverend MARTIN LUTHER KING JR.

A lot people say, "I'm personally opposed to abortion, but I think it should be legal. I don't have the right to force my beliefs and values on someone else." This is one of the most popular rationalizations for abortion. We've all heard this. This is at best a strange position to take because it is abstemious to an abnormal degree in democratic society. Most people don't morally abstain from other issues. This is a very common pro-choice argument, but it's a pro-choice argument with a twist. The person making this argument professes to have some reservations about abortion to start with, putting them on safer ground. It's just that this person doesn't want those reservations to change politics.

Many Democratic politicians used to make this kind of argument, even Hillary Clinton. This was frequently used by pro-choice politicians in order to win personal points, so that they don't sound like they're sanctioning the killing of innocent children. Rather, they want to sound empathetic to others by acknowledging that abortion is wrong while still being pro-choice and at the end of the day not changing their tune on the issue itself. It's almost as if they want all the moral credentials of being pro-life without having to actually be pro-life. How clever. Of course, Hillary Clinton and many Democrats who used to appear moderate in lip service by making these claims have since abandoned such arguments altogether; they now openly admit that they believe abortion is a positive good and something to be celebrated.[269] It is no longer lamented. How things have changed in this country—when Democrats don't even feel the need to hide their disdain for the unborn anymore.

But there are many others who genuinely feel this way who aren't political people. I have friends who think like this, who want their reservations to remain private. They are even reluctant to articulate these reservations, and they certainly don't want to pass laws that reflect these reservations. This is a curious argument because it denounces abortion while at the same time insisting that the speaker intends to take no steps to put that denunciation into action.

The argument was first popularly made in the 1980s when it was fashionable for religious Democrats to take refuge in this position. One of the most prominent exponents was New York Governor Mario Cuomo, father to the current governor of New York, Andrew Cuomo, and also to CNN host Chris Cuomo. Mario

Cuomo argued that he agreed with the Catholic Church on the fact that abortion is wrong. But he said as a politician, he was not going to impose that position on others. Geraldine Ferraro, a Democratic female vice presidential candidate, said in a 1984 debate, "I will accept the teaching of the church, but I cannot impose my religious views on someone else." She added, "I truly take an oath as a public official to represent all the people in my district, not only the Catholics."[270]

I can see how Christians fall into this trap, since Christians typically hate to impose their views on others. They would rather just tell themselves that they are taking the moral high road internally, but not feel the need to externally impose their views on others. "Christians have had the reputation of imposing their religion on others in history, so all the more reason for us Christians today to not act like this," a Christian might argue. The Christian who argues that he or she is "morally and personally opposed to the injustice of abortion, but would not impose their views on others" has mounted a moral high horse that has no foundation on which to stand. They somehow forget truth and send it to rest in the back of their mind, feeling perfectly good about this mental reconciliation.

Now, this position, or argument, might be called the "Pontius Pilate argument." Pontius Pilate was the Roman leader charged with hearing the case of none other than Jesus Christ himself. The accusations were made against Christ, and Pilate seemed to be leaning in favor of Jesus—yet he never puts that belief into action. Pilate says in effect: I wash my hands of this matter. In a sense Pilate was saying, I have reservations about the guilt of Jesus. I'm personally opposed to the idea of putting this man on a cross, sure. But I'm not going to impose my beliefs on others. I'm not going to carry it out politically. That's my personal view. (Sound familiar?)

So, Pilate then asks the crowd what they think. They yell that they want Jesus crucified. When Pilate asks them what Jesus has done, they can't say but merely repeat, "Crucify him!" Pilate, in order to appease the crowd, washes his hands, says, "I'm innocent of this man's blood, see to it yourselves," and delivers Jesus so that he can be crucified not by Pilate's hand, of course, but by guards and the rabble at large.

Just as Pilate was a decision maker in Rome, so are we decision makers in a democratic society. Obviously, we're not the decision makers in the sense that we sit on the Supreme Court. We might not be lawmakers. We might not be personally deciding to carry a pregnancy to term or to terminate it. But we are decision makers in the sense that we can campaign and we can vote. Those who use this "personally opposed to abortion" argument are doing far more than just passing the buck; they are supporting the pro-abortion side of the debate. How can they morally resolve such a position? Put simply, someone who is personally opposed to abortion but unwilling to impose their view on any other person is providing support for the whole gamut of pro-abortion activities.

The position being argued by people who don't want to impose their values on others is ultimately rooted in a kind of relativism. The view that these people really hold is not that they are pro-life but rather that their values are ultimately in the eye of the beholder. This is why one is reluctant to impose one's values. "They might be true for me, but they might not be true for you." Interestingly, Pontius Pilate himself was a kind of relativist. His famous line in the Bible is "What is truth?" and the very fact that he raises the question, not only in that way but phrased as a comeback, implies that Pilate is saying that truth is relative.

The position opposed to relativism goes back to the very beginning of Western civilization—the idea of what can be called natural right or natural law. Natural right is simply the idea that there is a moral order in the universe just as there is a physical order in the universe. There are certain things that are morally right and certain things that are morally wrong. In other words, the universe operates not only by physical or scientific laws but also by moral laws. While the physical and scientific laws tell us "this is the way things are," natural law tells us "this is the way things ought to be." And the core argument of natural right or natural law is the notion that even though there are different types of laws, physical laws and moral laws, they both have the status of truth.

Natural law and natural right, on the one hand, and relativism, on the other, are polar opposites and have been for centuries. This issue of absolute truth versus relativism was a hotly debated point at the beginning of Western civilization—even in Plato's *Republic*, where Socrates advocates natural right and the Sophists champion relativism. Socrates espouses the idea that there's such a thing as right and wrong in the world—and things are right or wrong in nature. One can believe that this distinction of right and wrong comes from God, or you can believe it is simply embedded in the moral order of the universe. But either way, it's there. Socrates has no doubt about it. But the Sophists say, nope, that's not true. They claim there's nothing that is right or wrong in nature—that things are right and wrong purely by custom.

People who don't want to impose their views on others are really saying they don't want to impose their beliefs on the woman, but they don't mind imposing their beliefs on the baby who is going to die because it seems customary to them. In other words, by pretending to be an innocent bystander, they sidestep the fact that their view has consequences no matter what and is going to result in an individual's death.

I want to be fair, though, to the innocent bystander, the person making this argument. What is the innocent bystander's obligation here? Bystanders who refuse to get involved in the life-and-death situation of another are only morally responsible to the degree that first, they know what's going on; second, that they have the power to do something about it; and third, whether it will cost them anything. No one is asking the bystander to physically jump in and stop someone else from getting an abortion. No one is asking the bystander to sacrifice their own life. But if you understand what is going on, you are being asked to do something that costs you literally nothing, which is cast your vote quietly in favor of life. And if you're willing to be bold, raise your voice and let the world know you are advocating for protecting life because then others will stand up, too. It's the least we can do for this cause, as this injustice continues in the country. The parable of the Good Samaritan, which is so often invoked, is not the case here in the sense that one does not need to jump in and give aid or to repel the attacker but merely to pull a lever in the voting booth. While this action costs you nothing, it can mean the difference in life or death for an innocent baby.

There is a great temptation in our culture, not just for Christians but for everyone, to not want to hurt anyone's feelings. To let everyone just live life, do as they please, and be happy. I get it; I don't want to hurt anyone's feelings either. I, too, want everyone to be happy. But when a moral injustice such as this looks you in the face, in this magnitude, in this real form, and is an important issue in question in our country at a time when you are living and able to participate, how can you be silent? We think that "being nice" means affirming everything—every worldview, every person's choice or opinion, no matter how harmful.

But how is it "nice" to others to mislead them by your silence into thinking that abortion on demand is morally acceptable? How is it "nice" to the baby who has to die? How is it "nice" to the woman who is puzzled by her pain afterward because everyone has been lying to her about what abortion really is and doesn't talk about it? We must wholeheartedly love others, and we must wholeheartedly oppose injustice as well. The two are not opposed. It is precisely because I love others that I cannot let injustice go on. We must never give up truth, for if we fall prey to relativism, then we have entered the gateway to evil.

Nobel Peace Prize winner and anti-apartheid preacher Desmond Tutu said, "If you are neutral in situations of injustice, you have chosen the side of the oppressor." There is no such thing as "not taking sides." There is no such thing as being "personally opposed." Your position is allowing the injustice to go on.

Those who claim to be "personally opposed" to abortion but don't want to impose this view on others are not actually that personally opposed to abortion in the first place, if at all. On the face of it, the "personally opposed" argument seems nuanced and heartfelt, but it quickly falls apart when you're talking about justifying killing other people. Abortion is wrong, not just "for you," not just "personally," but in itself. To justify the intentional killing of others means that you don't really think it's that evil.

CHAPTER FOURTEEN

MYTH: Abortion is never an ideal choice, but forcing a woman to carry out a pregnancy will cause her too much emotional pain. This is a situation only she can understand. I give preference to the woman, the person already here.

"Sir, you are giving a reason for it, but that will not make it right."

—SAMUEL JOHNSON in Boswell's *Life of Johnson*[271]

I want to consider an argument for the pro-choice position that marches behind the banner of realism. This argument concedes that abortion is an evil, but it's the lesser of two evils. It goes like this: there's something worse than an abortion, and that is destroying the emotional and personal life of the mother. This argument is typically made not by the woman having the abortion but by a third party defending the woman's right to have an abortion. People who make this argument usually say something along the lines of "We can't really understand what she's going through. We can't really fully grasp her situation. She'll make the best decision for her circumstances. Admittedly, she might have made decisions that have put her in this predicament, but we aren't perfect; people make mistakes. Women shouldn't have to live with a mistake. No one should be made to raise children against their will."

I hear this argument from friends in my everyday life as well as pundits and hosts of talk shows, like podcaster Dave Rubin, host of *The Rubin Report*, who has described himself in the past as "begrudgingly pro-choice."[272] I have also heard this from atheist Michael Shermer, editor of *Skeptic* magazine. These men argue that the fetus does have a claim to life, but they say that when weighing the claim of the fetus against the claim of the woman, the woman takes precedence. The argument is that the woman's life should be prioritized over the child's. They give the benefit to the person who was "here first." So, you have two lives pitted against each other, and they acknowledge that abortion is not ideal, but they believe that forcing the woman to go through emotional pain is bad. She may not be ready to cope with the pregnancy or with a child. After all, they say, she knows herself better than anyone. We must leave this up to her.

So, the woman's right not to be forced to complete her pregnancy has greater weight than the unspoken claim of the fetus to live. It reminds me of the old conundrum of two people in a lifeboat. The lifeboat is not strong enough to hold both. One person has to go overboard. It's not going to be easy, but you try to choose the lesser evil. It may seem shocking that pro-choice people compare life in this way. It seems like a heartless and crude utilitarian calculus. How can you really weigh the value of one life against another? We employ utilitarian calculus all the time, weighing one thing against another, and very often we assign numbers to these things. Maybe we rank how we are feeling on a scale of 1–10. We try to rank certain options in order to prioritize what we care about most, and this helps us make decisions and exercise personal preferences. But the problem with applying this type of utilitarian calculus to human life itself, or even to basic human dignity, is that it can lead to atrocious results.

Think, for example, of Aristotle's famous argument defending slavery. Aristotle acknowledges that slavery is a kind of injustice, but he argues that it's necessary. Why? He says that society needs it because there's dirty work to be done and someone has to do it. If you don't have people to do that kind of dirty work— the menial work, the sort of hard labor that is necessary to build a civilization—then you're not going to have a civilization that enables other people to be able to focus on contemplation or to pursue art or anything else involving higher culture and higher thinking. So, in this sense, slaves free up other people to take an interest in science and philosophy, which ultimately builds a better civilization. There's something chilling about his argument— an argument that stands on subjecting human dignity and human welfare, human life itself, to that kind of calculus and, ultimately, subjugation. When someone says, "I choose to side with the person already here," they are saying they choose the woman because if the child is aborted, then the woman is freed up to do other things. Favoring her, the argument might go, is better for society.

But this utilitarian comparison, often invoked by those who are pro-choice, is not a fair comparison. First, this is not a lifeboat situation where there are two people and only one can survive. There are instances where that would be the case, as in the case of a pregnancy with medical complications in which the fetus is a deadly threat to the life of the mother and there is no way both can survive. In that case, we are comparing one life with the life of another and making a valid comparison. It is quite different when we are talking about a pregnant woman who is perfectly healthy and are purely referring to her emotional state in coping with pregnancy. We're not in a "death-guaranteed scenario" where one party must die. We are not comparing the death of the mother, on the one hand, with the death of the fetus, on the other. We're comparing the emotional pain of the woman, on the one hand, with the death of the fetus, on the other. That's what's on each side of the scale.

We can all acknowledge that death is a far worse consequence than emotional pain. Everyone in human history has acknowledged this because whenever we're facing death, we try to avoid it. It's human nature to preserve our lives, no matter how horrendous the situation. Even if you're holding on to a rope on the side of a cliff, you're going to hold on to your life, despite all the pain you're in, in a herculean effort to save your life. Aside from the rare case of suicide, no one wants to die. And we know from those terrible ultrasound images of babies in the womb recoiling from the abortionist's death needle that even this tiny life instinctively reacts to danger.

Not Ready to Have a Child

But what about the woman whose reason for having an abortion is that she is not ready to have a child? This feeling is true of almost every woman, every couple, and every family. Because you're never truly ready to have a child until you have one. You're never ready to be a parent until you are one. Feeling like "I'm not really ready to have a child" makes complete sense because having a child is something that turns your world upside down. It changes your life forever. Most young parents aren't ready to take care of another human being. Most older parents aren't either. If you're young, maybe you have more energy, but you're also still figuring out your life. If you're older, you may be more financially stable and have a secure career, but you might not have as much time for child-rearing, be more set in your ways, and think a child would be exhausting and interfere in your life. The fact that someone doesn't feel ready to have a child doesn't mean that the child should die.

Keep in mind, most parents aren't ready to take care of their one-year-old, either, or their two-year-old. And many parents aren't emotionally capable of handling their teenagers either. People can't emotionally handle themselves sometimes, let alone another person. This is true of many of life's transitions, not just parenthood. No one is emotionally ready to hit middle age, for example. The loss of youth, the wrinkles, all of it is something that causes many older women emotional pain because their identity is so tied to how they saw themselves in their youth. We aren't ready for a lot of stages in life, but this doesn't warrant killing another person.

Every woman in America has the right to know that women have been sold a flat-out lie, which is that having an abortion is no big deal and that the emotions you feel after having an abortion will pass. But the reality is the opposite: the fear and feeling of "not being ready to have a child" are actually what will pass.

Empathy

A familiar refrain from the pro-choice side is "You could never understand her situation" or "None of us can understand what the woman is going through except her." Of course I agree that no one can fully understand any other person on Earth, in the sense of true and complete understanding, because we are not in fact that person and cannot physically and mentally be that person. Someone would best understand another who perhaps went through the same thing; however, they may only have that one experience in common and have many differences in other ways, including how they think about that common experience they share. But this does not mean we cannot relate to one another.

Humans have traditionally related to each other by showing empathy, which allows us to put ourselves in the shoes of another. We may not have experienced exactly what someone else has experienced, but we've experienced something that has generated a similar emotion. For example, if you have lost a parent, this may clearly help you relate to someone else who has also lost a parent, but that experience of pain and the loss of someone dear and familiar may also allow you to relate to others in pain because they lost their child, their childhood friend, their home, or something else that had great meaning for them. You may empathize with someone who feels left out of a certain friend group because there have been times when you felt unwelcome or uninvited or excluded, albeit in different circumstances. We can all relate to human emotions, even if we experienced them due to a different catalyst. Loss and pain are things we all understand through different experiences.

Experience and empathy allow us to have a sense of what something else feels like, even if we don't know exactly what another person is going through and they haven't even shared all of the information with us. If a woman is having a difficult time with an unexpected pregnancy, I agree that it's impossible for us to have complete knowledge of her innermost thoughts combined with the way she was raised, where she is living and working, what her relationships are like, and all of the things that have come together to make her the person she is.

But we often do not need to have full knowledge or complete understanding of another person's situation to be able to look at the information we do have and take meaningful action to alleviate it. When we say, "I know how you feel," we really don't know entirely, but we know enough to motivate us to take action.

Whenever the emotional pain argument is invoked in the case of abortion, it often only applies to the woman. Maybe you have not had an abortion yourself, but maybe you have been through a situation that you didn't think you could handle or cope with. Maybe you have even been through an unwanted pregnancy. Maybe one of your children was a surprise. Maybe you have had the feeling of it being too much to bear. But none of us has been the one to be killed. None of us can truly understand what it's like to have someone target your heart and pierce it with a needle that will kill you or be suctioned through a vacuum. When we empathize, we must remember to empathize with both the woman and the fetus. There are incredible survivors of abortion (babies who lived through it), but most of us have not experienced it. Ironically, this makes it easier for us to empathize with the woman in a difficult situation because we have all been through difficult situations but harder for us to empathize with the targeted fetus. Most of us have not been brutally targeted and maimed or killed. But this does not mean we should not care. The victims of the Holocaust, the survivors of immense torture and pain, as well as the unborn babies in the womb, the most vulnerable in our society today, are people we must attempt to understand. When we see their pain, we need to try to empathize, even if we have not experienced it, and ultimately stop it.

Emotional Pain

So, what about the emotional pain of a woman with an unwanted pregnancy? The problem when we hear this argument is that it examines one type of emotional pain—the emotional pain of having a child—but doesn't compare it to its counterpart, which is the emotional pain of having the abortion itself. Let's compare adoption and abortion, since those are the two options women typically consider in the case of a truly unwanted pregnancy. Should anyone be forced to raise a child against their will? Of course not. No one is forced to because there's always the beautiful option of adoption.

Frederica Mathewes-Green, a writer and former pro-choice feminist herself, wrote, "No one wants an abortion as she wants an ice cream cone or a Porsche. She wants an abortion as an animal, caught in a trap, wants to gnaw off its own leg."[273] Many women who get an abortion choose to do so because they feel they have no other option. Abortion clinics everywhere do a terrible and dishonest service to frightened women who are in a desperate situation and looking for answers by not promoting adoption more. Some women don't even know how to go about giving their child up for adoption because clinics don't bring it up. If you go into a Planned Parenthood looking for answers, they will not counsel you on adoption options. They just offer the abortion.

When it comes to abortion, many women tell themselves they just want to get in there, get it done, get it over with, and forget it ever happened. But this is nothing more than the memory trying to erase itself, almost as if through consumption of alcohol or drugs to numb oneself and blot out reality. Of course, memory doesn't disappear in this convenient way. It stays with many women for the rest of their lives, even when they don't want it to.

If you take away another person's life, if you become their judge, jury, and executioner, that is going to be a source of deep, emotional pain, far more emotional pain than if you had birthed the child and given it up for adoption. If you know that you are choosing the death of your child intentionally and directly for your own benefit, just think of the emotional burden you will bear for making that choice. And I know many women live for the rest of their lives with this shameful skeleton in their past. It is purely tragic.

At least after nine months of pregnancy, you can know that in giving up the baby for adoption, it is going to people who want the child. Even if those nine months are the worst of your entire life and you truly believe you are enduring deep emotional suffering, this will likely produce less emotional pain for you than killing the child. Socrates says it is better to suffer wrong than to do wrong because the "doing-wrong" harms your soul. If you are not the wrongdoer, at least you can rest easy in knowing that you made the merciful decision. When we look at women who have given their child up for adoption, almost none would say they wish they had aborted it. Some would say they wish they had kept it, but never aborted it.

Of course, the Left tries to deflect attention away from this. They love to celebrate abortions, to parade women who have had abortions, women who say they feel completely happy about it, and portray it as a purely logical decision. This kind of propaganda, pushed by the media, is an attempt to normalize the procedure to women who haven't had one, and it is intended to silence the sense of regret experienced by women who have had one. The little voice inside that says, "This is not something I should have done. I could have carried the baby to term and given up for adoption. Instead, I carried it to the grave." This sentiment is something the Left will never acknowledge; they will never print it in any piece they run on abortion.

As a result of this lie, the emotional toll associated with abortion is often buried deep or hidden behind closed doors. The Left doesn't want to talk about women who suffer emotionally from abortion because they don't want anyone to think too much about what abortion actually is. If you do suffer emotionally, the Left will say that's just your personal feeling and it doesn't bear any weight on the issue itself. It doesn't change a woman's "right to choose."

Is it ethical for abortion doctors to lead women through those doors and into that operating room without explaining the emotional toll of the procedure? Abortion doctors send women home—women who leave the abortion clinic not just in physical pain but with a deeper sense of emotional pain that something has been lost, something you can never get back. This is far too much of a burden for one person to bear alone. And for the media and the abortion industry to be working in tandem to mislead women is truly an atrocity.

This is why we must console and help women heal from abortion because so much hurt is left behind. So many amazing pro-life women help others heal through organizations like Sisters of Life and Focus on the Family. While the Left does not accept women who deeply regret having had an abortion, we love them and welcome them into our hearts and homes with open arms. We have all made mistakes in life and are no better than anyone who has made this particular mistake. We have all been through deep pain, regret, and loss. While the life lost can never be brought back, love and purpose can surely be restored in the woman who struggles with this.

A woman who finds herself pregnant and unable to fathom caring for a baby thinks about abortion versus adoption. While they both provide an answer, these two options have entirely different results. While abortion leads to death for the child, adoption results in life. Abortion takes the woman's current situation, already difficult, and makes it worse by leaving her emotionally scarred. Adoption allows for light at the end of the tunnel and for a solution for both mother and child. While abortion is punitive and involves permanent loss, adoption is redemptive and allows for the child to have a better life. If we think about both situations, abortion and adoption, they both tug on the heartstrings and are emotionally difficult for the mother. I do not deny this. Even if we put aside the difficulty of abortion, adoption isn't easy. It takes strength to give up your child to another family and to say goodbye. In both situations you are separating from your child. But taking away the child's life is entirely different than giving it a better life. At least in sending it to a family that will care for it, you know it is in good hands.

If we think about what love really means, it is that you wish the best for the other person. Love isn't "I feel happy around this person" or seeing a person as serving your needs. Love isn't merely a fleeting feeling but a decision to put the other person first. Love is sacrificial in that you genuinely put that other person's welfare above your own and want to see them happy. Maybe you're a teen mom, maybe you need to finish school, or maybe you are older but just know that you can't care for the child. The most sacrificial thing you can do is to put your child in the arms of a family who will give it that love and care that you know it deserves.

I have a good friend who is adopted. She has known she was adopted ever since she was a kid. She's grateful that her birth mother gave her up for adoption. She was adopted by remarkable people, a couple who raised her and understands that her birth mother was not in a position to do the same. She now has a relationship with her birth mother, although distant, but she views her birth mother as somewhat of a hero. Why? Because her birth mother had the option to abort but chose not to. My friend is grateful that her mom chose to give her a loving home instead of ending her life. My friend is a smart woman. She has a great job. She loves her family that raised her, that she has grown up with all her life. And there's no doubt that she's happy she is alive rather than being dead. She is grateful every day because her mother chose life.

Adoption is a form of love because it involves self-sacrifice. Whenever we look at situations of adoption, we see that many people were putting thought into this child: the mother who chose to have the child and sought out a plan for its future, the adoption agency or organization that facilitated the process, and the family that adopted the child and awaited its arrival. So we see that lots of love and thought were poured into this child and its welfare.

The fact that there are thirty-six families waiting to adopt a child for every one child available shows that there is a vast desire for adoption.[274] While abortion is on demand, adoption is at least a yearlong process. It's sad that adoptive parents wait so long to adopt a child, hoping that a mother picks them. In the end, many of these parents never get to adopt because there is such a shortage of children being given up for adoption. The CDC states that over 57 percent of families that struggle with fertilization treatments consider adoption.[275] This doesn't take into account the many families that are seeking to adopt not due to infertility but due to a desire to grow their family or other reasons. Families seeking to adopt undergo financial, criminal, and medical background checks. Their home is subject to inspection. Mothers can often handpick the family they want to give the baby to, look through countless profiles of the families in need, meet them, and interview them. They can make another family's dreams come true. If organizations like Planned Parenthood were truly focused on "parenthood" as their name suggests, as well as women's health, then they should be promoting adoption instead of performing abortions.

In sum, abortion is not the lesser of two evils. Whether it is due to inconvenience or insurmountable emotional pain, a woman who does not want her child does not have to choose between raising it and killing it. Adoption is a beautiful option because you allow the child to be raised by someone else who desperately wants it, intends to give it the best care, and is willing to do so. Let yourself make this decision with the full knowledge that you did what is best for your child, spare yourself the emotional pain of abortion, and then go forth with gratitude.

CHAPTER FIFTEEN

MYTH: Outlawing abortion doesn't decrease the number of abortions. It merely forces the process underground, leading to back-alley abortions like in the old days.

> "There is not a crime, there is not a dodge, there is not a trick, there is not a swindle, there is not a vice which does not live by secrecy."
>
> —JOSEPH PULITZER

The pro-choice argument for abortion relies not only on philosophical claims but also on a historical narrative they've created that proceeds from the "bad old days" of the past to a more enlightened present. It is presented as a story of progress. In this view, things used to be terrible, and they got better because of abortion, so to regulate, restrict, or abolish abortion is to go back to the bad old days. Therefore, the pro-choice position is promoted as inherently progressive and enlightened, while the pro-life position is scorned as unenlightened and reactionary. The Left has tried hard to push the narrative that women were risking their lives to get abortions before *Roe v. Wade*. For example, Senator Diane Feinstein tweeted in January 2020: "Today's the 47th anniversary of *Roe v. Wade*. I remember the days before *Roe*, when women risked their lives so they could make their own decisions about their health care. We can't return to those dark days. I'm more committed than ever to protecting a woman's right to choose."[276]

Safe, Legal, and Rare

The Clintons liked to say that abortions should be "safe, legal, and rare" when Bill Clinton was president. But the "safe, legal, and rare" slogan doesn't actually make any sense. The question we must ask ourselves is—Why should it be rare? If there is nothing wrong with aborting a child and it is merely a health procedure, why should it be rare? Why shouldn't it be treated like any other medical procedure where it is just safe and legal? The fact that one thinks it should be rare reveals the recognition that one knows that what we have here is, in fact, a child, a human being who is going to be killed in the process—and that is regrettable and should be "rare." You can't say that abortion should be rare and also say the baby is not a person.

Law Affects Behavior

By making something legal, it inherently becomes more common because people think it is okay and can obtain it easily. This is the case with abortion. We have seen over sixty-one million abortions— sixty-one million babies killed since 1973. That is not "rare." According to the National Institutes of Health, the primary agency of the U.S. government responsible for public health research, about half of women going in for abortion procedures have had one before.[277] The repeat abortion rate, at around 50 percent, has tripled since it stood at 15 percent in 1974.[278] This indicates that many women are using abortion as a form of birth control.

Conversely, by making something illegal, it statistically becomes rarer. Realistically, anytime something is made difficult to get, fewer people get it. Consider prohibition laws, which were reviled and flouted but still decreased instances of drinking. Even after drinking was permitted again, the issues of violent alcoholism didn't return to the degree they had existed before. And keep in mind that this law was incredibly difficult to enforce, since people could easily drink in their own home. And yet even this was effective. It is a law of economics and human nature that laws and restrictions affect behavior. If you want to reduce the instance of a certain action, you have to make it illegal. Every criminal code is based on this principle. Yet, when it comes to the single issue of abortion, the principle is denied.

The way to really prevent back-alley abortions is to pursue and prosecute abortionists. If abortions were made illegal, the number of people willing to perform abortions illegally would vastly decrease. This would also save the innocent lives of babies and prevent women from being put through unsafe and unregulated medical procedures. A pro-choicer might say: If abortion were illegal throughout America, would you really prosecute women who abort their babies as murderers? The law would focus on the abortion doctors themselves. Just as the government doesn't focus on drug users but drug dealers and focuses on busting pimps, not prostitutes. You prosecute the professional, not the client. You prosecute the people doing this systematically, which is clearly the abortion doctor.

In *The Demoralization of Society: From Victorian Virtues to Modern Values*, Gertrude Himmelfarb writes, "You cannot legislate morality, it is often said. Yet we have done just that. Civil rights legislation prohibiting racial discrimination has succeeded in proscribing racist conduct not only legally but morally as well."[279] This goes to show that changing people's hearts and minds so that abortion is inconceivable goes hand in hand with it being illegal. Those two goals are not mutually exclusive. It is not a matter of either-or but both-and.

Leftists argue that if abortion is illegal, the number of abortions will be the same, but they will be unsafe back-alley abortions. This is actually not true. The number of maternal deaths resulting from back-alley abortions "in the old days" is heavily exaggerated. According to the CDC, in 1972, the year before *Roe v. Wade*, there were thirty-nine maternal deaths due to back-alley abortions.[280] However, pro-abortion organizations like the National Abortion Rights Action League (NARAL) claimed to document "the real numbers" when it came to back-alley abortion statistics, declaring that thousands of women were dying per year due to back-alley abortions. It did this in order to tug on the heartstrings of Americans hearing these numbers.

But in 1979, a powerful man admitted to forging those numbers—his name is Dr. Bernard Nathanson. He cofounded NARAL, personally oversaw over sixty-five thousand abortions, and performed five thousand abortions himself. He is a credible person on this issue and had the power to validate the numbers on this. In his book *Aborting America*, he wrote, "How many deaths were we talking about when abortion was illegal? In NARAL...it was always 5,000 to 10,000 deaths....I confess that I knew the figures were totally false."[281] This is something that pro-choice activists and the media do not want you to hear. We know what the actual numbers were. So, the truth is that back-alley abortions are not nearly as common as people on the Left would like you to believe, and neither are maternal deaths due to back-alley abortions. Even Planned Parenthood concedes that there were fewer than five hundred women who died per year due to back-alley abortions prior to *Roe v. Wade*.[282]

While the Left constantly harks back to "coat hanger abortions" to represent back-alley abortions prior to the 1970s, there are a few back-alley abortions that go on today, even when abortion is legal. When *Vox* comes out with articles like "Self-Managed Abortion Is Medically Very Safe," *Cosmopolitan* publishes articles like "Should Women Perform Their Own Abortions?" and *Hub Culture* gives the advice "7 Effective and Risk-Free Home Remedies for Abortion," the idea of aborting your own baby at home is gaining traction and cultural currency.[283] Women don't use coat hangers anymore but instead opt for "wellness" techniques like special teas and aerobic movements. This may seem shocking, but it is going on within the pro-choice world of the Left, with media messaging to support it. It almost seems like they are anticipating an end to *Roe v. Wade*.

Inga Muscio, pro-choice speaker and writer, tells us about her three abortions in her book *Cunt: A Declaration of Independence*. After having two painful surgical abortions, she decided to have the third abortion at home. She used naturopathic techniques from a friend she calls simply "Judy," who came to her house every night to perform what she calls "an incantation."[284] She says it took eight days of drinking teas with special concoctions and performing intense movements at home in order to reach the moment of abortion. She says, "I was brushing my teeth at the sink and felt a very peculiar mmmmbloommmp-like feeling. I looked at the bathroom floor and there, between my feet, was some blood and a little round thing. It was clear but felt like one of them unshiny superballs....It was the neatest thing I ever did see. An orb of life and energy, in my hand...I wore black for a week and had a little funeral in my head."[285] She concludes, "My cuntlovin friends and I did something amazing to affect my destiny in the most conducive way possible."[286]

While her story is disturbing, to say the least, and she surely represents a small and strange subculture of the population, the point is this: at-home back-alley abortions go on today, even while abortion is legal. If the pro-choice side acts like back-alley abortions are their worst nightmare, why are they promoting them and doing them in this glorified at-home fashion?

If abortion was illegal throughout the United States, I suspect the following would happen: a few people, like Inga Muscio, would perform mind boggling at-home abortion rituals, but anyone like that who would do so later is doing so already. Condoms and other forms of contraception would be of the utmost importance to people who don't want to have children. Abortion pills that work up to ten weeks into pregnancy would become like underground drugs. Any abortion performed after ten weeks would become rare because suction, D&C, and induction abortion are all surgeries that require anesthesia and medical devices, and at that point they would only be performed by quacks. Many women would not want to put themselves through an unregulated procedure like that.

One might retort, "Okay, if *Roe v. Wade* were overturned and if abortion were illegal nationwide due to a constitutional amendment, people could just leave the country to get it." True. All kinds of things happen in other countries that we don't allow here.

People can currently go to other countries to get drugs that aren't FDA-approved. Laws passed in America don't apply to other countries because other countries have their own sets of laws. The fact that people would have to leave the country in order to get an abortion is the most we can limit it, but it's definitely a hurdle worth putting in place because it is a deterrent. Anytime someone has to leave the country, it is expensive and time-consuming. The Left would say that this only inhibits poor people, but that's not true. Even for a wealthy person it would be complicated because there is also timing when it comes to pregnancy, so every week that passes means you are further along.

Additionally, many countries don't have abortion laws as liberal as the ones we currently have here; so, for example, if you wanted a third-trimester abortion in most countries in Europe, you wouldn't be able to get one unless for a medical reason. America is currently a country with some of the most pro-abortion laws in the world, comparable to Russia and China. So, if you wanted an abortion late-term, you'd have to head to one of those countries. A macabre site would be abortion tourism. Of course, there are ways around the logistics, and someone like George Soros, a big funder of pro-abortion activity, could bankroll women's flights to get abortions outside America. There are so many radical leftists who advocate for killing, I wouldn't be surprised. We cannot regulate the laws of other countries, just our own. In fact, it is our responsibility to do so.

CHAPTER SIXTEEN

MYTH: Abortion is necessary because of hard cases like rape, incest, life of the mother, and potential medical complications. No parent should be forced to have a deformed or mentally challenged child. None of us would want to be in that position.

"I am a man with Down syndrome and my life is worth living."[287]

—FRANK STEPHENS, human rights advocate

It is commonly said that hard cases make bad law. Yet in discussions of law and policy, hard cases are frequently invoked. Why is this? The reason is hard cases appeal to emotion—never more so than for the advocates of the pro-life cause. Some people with pro-life sympathies are quick to concede the hard cases. They point out that hard cases are exceptional and a significant minority of the overall cases under discussion. Therefore, by excluding them from the debate and conceding them, it makes the debate easier to win. This is not my approach. I will meet the hard cases head-on and argue that we should strive for life in all circumstances—with no exceptions, realizing that it may not be possible in all circumstances.

People who want to debate me on abortion love to discuss the hard cases. *They love to!* They use these cases as a starting point to say that because there are hard cases, abortion should be available in all cases. No one who invokes the hard cases says—Let's only allow abortion in these hard cases. No, they invoke hard cases in order to justify all abortions. They want you to be on the slippery slope. This logic needs to be resisted. When I discuss hard cases, I am only referring to hard cases, and my arguments settle nothing outside these.

Childbirth in America used to be much more dangerous than it is today. Women frequently died in childbirth in the eighteenth and nineteenth centuries. In the Civil War era, for example, a woman might have been hemorrhaging and near death, but this didn't mean doctors knew how to save either the woman or the child. Sometimes both the woman and child died in the childbirth process, sometimes only the woman, and sometimes only the child. The situation of comparing lives in equal danger did not arise often, and realistically doctors and midwives could not usually control who died but would do the best they could in the moment to salvage the situation.

A woman might yell something in the moment like, "Save my baby! Not me!" because there is such a strong bond between mother and child, and mothers at that time shared a deep belief that sacrificing your child for your own benefit was wrong. The doctor could listen but not always control whom he could save. If in doubt about which life to "save first," I think the doctor should always choose to save the mother first because the child is still living in her as well, so saving her first would be best for both parties. This certainly does not mean you are killing the child.

This debate shows how times have changed, how social mores and values have changed, and how the abortion debate is quite different from what we see here. If I were to tell a radical leftist that in cases where the life of the mother is in danger, it would be understandable for a doctor to save the woman first and then the child, they would probably spit in my face and call me a "radical" and "anti-woman" because to them the obvious answer is to kill the baby immediately. We must love them both, the woman and the child. And saving both should be the outcome we strive for in a medical emergency.

Initially, arguments for abortion in America only applied to specific circumstances. Historically, situations that involved severe deformities and other special circumstances were drawn to the forefront of the debate. While these occurrences were clearly rare, occurring less than 1 percent of the time, abortions were granted in these special cases. But, without question, it was these decisions that eventually opened the floodgates for abortion due to "emotional health" and "general health." Abortion was deemed necessary to preserve not just the woman's physical life but her emotional life as well. This turned into "abortion on demand" and abortion at nine months for no medical reason. Abortion without a medical reason is the America in which we are living today.

It is important to keep in mind that the entire debate about whether hard cases, like the life of the mother, rape, incest, and deformed children, warrant abortion is not politically relevant at this moment in American history. Democrats do not even argue that life should be protected in all circumstances except these. They argue that perfectly healthy children, who have no deformities, with mothers with no medical complications, who were not conceived in rape or incest, can die on demand, too. We are not at a point in American history where abortion is illegal throughout the country and we are trying to seriously discuss exceptions. We are at a point in American history where abortion on demand for no reason is the norm, and any rollback, including heartbeat bills and attempts to limit third-trimester, that is, late-term abortion, is seen as anti-woman and reactionary.

The pro-life battle we are fighting is far off from this chapter, which deals with hard cases. So, we must remind ourselves that debates confined to this chapter are essentially intellectual exercises. The only reason the pro-choice side likes to invoke "hard cases" is because leftists secretly know that pro-life people are sympathetic to both mothers and their children, and they also know that we are not wicked people. If they thought we were so wicked, they would not bother bringing up hard cases at all, since it wouldn't work to appeal to anyone's emotions. And they love to go here because it puts us on the defense and them on the offense.

Let's look at the "life of the mother." The argument used to be that abortion could only be performed for serious life-and-death medical reasons. If *Roe v. Wade* were overturned, doctors would still be able to save the life of the mother. Doctors are freely able to save the life of the mother now, and they were also freely able to do so before *Roe v. Wade*. Doctors have always been instructed by the law to save the woman's life, even if that means not being able to also save the fetus. But I think what is helpful here is to dive into specific types of threats to the mother's life so that we can think more deeply about these situations.

Pregnant Cancer Patients

Let's look at the case of the pregnant cancer patient. This is a difficult case because it is a life-threatening situation for both the mother and child. This is a debate discussed among the medical community, as well as scholars of ethics, because when a woman who has cancer gets pregnant or a pregnant woman suddenly gets cancer, we are faced with a dilemma: chemotherapy, radiation, other surgeries, and anesthesia performed on a pregnant woman with cancer can harm the baby. The baby is most vulnerable and affected by these treatments in the first trimester. With highly aggressive cancers, like acute leukemia, some lymphomas, and breast cancer, early aggressive therapy can be essential and the difference between life and death for the woman. In cancers that are not highly aggressive, sometimes doctors are able to circumvent the issue by postponing treatment until the baby has reached the second or third trimester, when there is less likelihood that treatment will affect the child. Ideally, they are able to wait until after the baby is born. While the precision of modern radiation therapy has improved, there is still a chance that the baby could be negatively affected by it.[288]

So, the woman is faced with a choice: abort the child and receive cancer treatment, let the child continue to develop and receive cancer treatment, or let the child continue to develop and wait to receive cancer treatment. Many Christians, especially Catholics, think about this situation and employ what is called, "the principle of double effect." The principle dates back to Thomas Aquinas and states that double effect occurs when an action is followed by two effects, one effect that is good and intended and one effect that is bad and unintended but foreseen.[289] The principle is that it is morally permissible to perform an action when the deed itself is morally good or neutral as long as the intention is the positive outcome and the negative outcome is a side effect. Taking this action that has the positive effect as well as the negative side effect should be the last resort as well. This principle states that it is completely different to directly bring about the negative outcome.

In this situation that would mean that if a woman had uterine cancer, it would be morally permissible for her to have a hysterectomy, removing the cancer (the positive intended outcome), even if the death of the fetus results as the negative unintended outcome of the cancer being removed. Aborting the child on purpose is completely different because that is a direct action taken with the intention to kill. We must remember that it is not the child that is the cancer, so removing the cancer is acceptable and directly killing the child is not.

Ethical thinkers have thought about dilemmas such as this for years, even before the issue of pregnant cancer patients arose. Just war theory draws on this logic as well. Just war theory states that it is permissible to target military, commanding forces, and the other side's army who are fighting you, but it is not morally permissible to directly target civilians. It would be completely different to target a military base and accidentally kill civilians that are on the military base than it would be to directly target civilians on purpose. Regardless of whether you agree with this moral theory, the point is that we should strive to protect innocent life.

Medical Complications in Pregnancy

There are medical complications when it comes to pregnancy. Famed opera singer Andrea Bocelli once told this story: "A young pregnant wife has been hospitalized for a simple attack of appendicitis. The doctors had to apply ice to her stomach and when the treatments ended, the doctors suggested that she abort the child. They told her it was the best solution because the baby would be born with some disability, but the young, brave wife decided not to abort, and the child was born. That woman was my mother, and I was the child."[290] Although Bocelli is blind, he has blessed the world by opening our eyes to the truth and beauty he expresses in his testimony and his voice.

The mother of Tim Tebow, the American football star, was asked in an interview what time in her life was the hardest and she said that it was when she was pregnant with Tim. While serving as a missionary with her husband in the Philippines, she contracted severe amoebic dysentery, usually caused by contaminated drinking water. She fell into a coma and was treated with strong drugs to combat the infection. It was then discovered that she was pregnant. She was told by doctors that the drugs likely caused the fetus severe placental abruption, meaning the placenta detached from the uterine wall, depriving the fetus' brain of oxygen. She explained, "I was told to abort him, and I didn't. The doctor said that I could lose my life if I didn't and we didn't have good medical care because we were living in an area of the Philippines." But she chose to have him anyway because of her faith in God. In an interview, Tim Tebow once told of how supportive his siblings were of his birth: "They thought I was a tumor and so when I was born and old enough to remember, they always called me Timmy the Tumor," he said with a chuckle.[291] Tim Tebow, famous for being an NFL player who is also a pro-life Christian, appeared in a Super Bowl ad put out by Focus on the Family that had a pro-life message, telling the story of him and his mom and how he came to be born. He was criticized for it heavily by pro-choice advocates.

Ectopic pregnancy is an instance in which the woman's life is in danger. This is when a fertilized egg is implanted outside the main cavity of the uterus where it is supposed to be, usually in a fallopian tube. An egg in this position cannot survive without threatening the mother's life, and if left untreated the growing fetus will cause bleeding and the rupture of the fallopian tube, leaving the fetus unable to continue development and the mother at risk of death.[292] Ectopic pregnancy is rare, occurring about 1 percent of the time in pregnancy. This percentage increases if you are a woman who has undergone IVF (infertility treatment), increasing the risk of ectopic pregnancy to 4 percent. Those who are chronic smokers, those with sexually transmitted infections, and those who become pregnant with an IUD in place are also at a greater risk of experiencing ectopic pregnancy.[293] If you are none of these things, your chance of having an ectopic pregnancy is even lower than 1 percent.

There are instances where ectopic pregnancies can be monitored closely at a hospital and the baby can be delivered at twenty-eight weeks.[294] Autotransfusion, where the woman receives her own blood in a transfusion, is a more effective method than abortion to save the life of the mother, since blood loss is the primary threat to the mother's life and this replaces the blood.[295] Most doctors do not take the approach of trying to save both the mother and the baby and instead opt for an early abortion for the baby. Despite the haste to kill, there are stories of babies and their mothers who both survive ectopic pregnancy.

After being encouraged to abort, one woman with an ectopic pregnancy said, "Paul and I agreed that as long as I was in no immediate danger, we would continue for as long as possible to give the baby a fighting chance. Now we can't believe we have such a beautiful, healthy, and happy little girl—it's a miracle."[296]

Another problem with immediately aborting ectopic pregnancies is that many are misdiagnosed. "Despite advances in medical imaging, roughly 40 percent of pregnancies diagnosed as ectopic are later revealed to be normal, intrauterine pregnancies."[297] Dr. Yaron Finkelstein, an emergency physician at Sick Kids Hospital and associate professor of pharmacology and toxicology at the University of Toronto, says, "This is a serious problem, and one that's probably overlooked."[298]

Preeclampsia, if left untreated, can be life-threatening. Preeclampsia usually occurs after twenty weeks and affects about 5 percent of pregnancies. The condition causes high blood pressure and typically goes away within weeks of giving birth.[299] It is something that can be monitored closely by a doctor, with bed rest and medicine to lower blood pressure. The only cure is delivery, which will be induced early if the woman is near term. About 15 percent of babies are born early because of preeclampsia.[300]

There are other instances of complications in pregnancy—many of which are common and not life-threatening. For example, many women develop an ovarian cyst during pregnancy, which can be uncomfortable but typically disappears in the second trimester without intervention. Ovarian cysts can be monitored with ultrasound.[301] Sometimes the woman develops serious back pain. A woman who has had a miscarriage in the past is under increased risk of a miscarriage happening again. But that doesn't mean you need to induce an abortion.

There are women who we know will have high-risk pregnancies before they even get pregnant. This is the case for women older than thirty-five and more so if you are older than forty. This is also true for women who are obese or already have HIV/AIDS, high blood pressure, or diabetes.[302] As a result, diabetes is monitored, blood pressure is lowered, and if the woman has AIDS, she will take medication that that will protect the baby.[303]

Jumping on the "life-of-the-mother" argument, the Left began to argue for the woman's emotional life—claiming that her emotional state was at stake. This is when the floodgates opened. This is a common argument used by those on the Left because this exception seems to give them grounds to allow abortion for any reason. I discuss this in more depth in a different chapter. The pro-choicers say they "don't want a doctor's hands to ever be tied." Bottom line: a doctor's hands should be tied when it comes to killing a child without cause.

In Cases of Rape

Now let's shift to discussing a different hard case—pregnancies resulting from rape. It is estimated that less than one-half of 1 percent of abortions involve victims of rape, according to the Guttmacher Institute.[304] Before even getting into this hard case, we should all know that the way to prevent children from being conceived in rape is to vigorously prosecute rapists and keep them off the streets.

For me, there is nothing inconsistent about being pro-life and pro-death penalty. I like what Kelsey Grammar said: "If someone has to die as a result of rape, then we should kill the rapist—not the unborn child."[305] Regardless of your view of the death penalty, if anyone should get the death penalty it certainly shouldn't be the innocent child. If Democrats can't see that a rapist is different from an innocent baby, they are morally blind.

Two Wrongs Don't Make a Right

So, then what about the debate of whether abortion is justified in the case of rape? The woman has been horribly violated. Her rights have been completely taken away from her by this rapist. But

what is abortion if not violating the rights of another in such a brutal fashion as sucking out their brains and breaking their bones? I
don't think piling two wrongs on top of each other makes a right.
No woman deserves to be violated. If a woman who is raped is
pregnant and there is no way we can rewind time to where she
wasn't raped in the first place, then what is the best thing to do
going forward from this situation? I don't think it's to kill the child.
The Left sees killing the child as a form of "rewinding time," but it
doesn't. The result is a dead child.

Oftentimes, children conceived in rape are a reminder of the
rapist, and it can be too painful for the woman to endure seeing it.
This is completely understandable. The mother can give the child
up for adoption. Closed adoptions are where the mother and child
never have contact and neither will be able to know what happened to the other. Another family will love the baby and not see
it in that light. Obviously, the child is better off being loved rather
than killed.

While the woman may never forget the rape, she also may never
forget getting an abortion. The emotional pain she is going through
at this time will not disappear because of the abortion. She will
now be carrying two painful memories: one that was not her choice
and one that was. That's an incredibly painful place to be in.

Another problem with arguing that women should be able to
abort their baby if raped is that it won't just be women who were
raped coming in for abortions. Many women will lie about being
raped, who were not actually raped, just so they can get an abortion. This will result in men being wrongfully convicted, and making this false claim could become the norm after every unwanted
pregnancy.

Actor Martin Sheen relates to this issue personally because his wife, Janet, was conceived in rape. Her mother could have aborted her but chose not to. Sheen says that Janet's mother contemplated "dumping her in the Ohio River." Janet was then raised by aunts until she was six, after which her mother "came to collect her."[306] Sheen and Janet have been married since 1961. He knows that if Janet's mother had aborted her, she would not be alive today.

Pregnant Children

About 0.3 percent of abortions are done on girls fifteen years old or younger. What about when children are pregnant? I see this in the same light as rape because children are not able to give legal consent. Incest with a minor is the same because minors can't give consent. When minors are pregnant, we should return to the first section of this chapter, regarding the life of the mother. If a child who has not reached puberty is pregnant, her life is at great risk, and no matter what your age is, the life of the mother should always be preserved.

The youngest person to give birth was a girl in Peru who was raped at age five and gave birth at age six. Her parents didn't know she was pregnant, so they took her to the hospital thinking she had a tumor on her stomach. She was actually seven months pregnant. She delivered via cesarean section, and her brother raised the baby.[307] It was discovered that she was able to get pregnant at that age because she had a rare case of precocious puberty. She went on to grow up, work, and have another child when she was older, and she is still alive at age eighty-six. I bring this up to point out that there are perverts out there who would rape a five-year-old girl. There are even such sick people out there who do this to babies, literally with an umbilical cord. It is sickening to think that anyone could do this, but this furthers my point about why we must stop these sick rapists.

Incest

Less than 0.01 percent of abortions are due to incest, according to reports from the CDC in Florida. (Not all states are required to report.)[308] This is the rarest of all of the hard cases we have discussed. When it comes to consensual incest among adults, there is no excuse, and I have no sympathy. They chose to engage in this action, and that is disgusting as well as illegal. You can't marry your brother or sister. Both adults should be prosecuted for this. Incest is extremely rare, but again, the action is not the fault of the child. The child, just as any other child, including children with disabilities as I will discuss next, should be loved and cared for.

"No Parent Should Be Forced to Have a Deformed or Mentally Challenged Child. None of Us Would Want to Be in That Position."

I now want to shift to discuss the next hard case brought up by pro-choicers, which is children with disabilities. I would like to begin by saying that there are many babies who were supposed to have a medical problem or some sort of abnormality, and the doctor explained that the child might be at risk, but in the end the baby was fine. There are limits to what doctors know and likelihood doesn't mean that something is definitely going to happen. And even if it is 100 percent certain that the child is going to come into this world with medical or mental issues, we cannot take its life because of this. It is still a person, and it's still a life. Some may ask what kind of life it is. And the bottom line is, it is in every way a life. When you get to know children with Autism, Down syndrome, you name it, it's easy to see they experience emotions and live full lives. They are people, too. As soon as we become killers of the disadvantaged, or anyone who is different from us, we become eugenicists.

A leftist might say, "Many parents who have mentally challenged children wouldn't say it, but they clearly wish they didn't. If they could do it over differently, certainly they would. Children with Down syndrome suck the life out of the parents and are physically, mentally, and financially exhausting for them. Mentally challenged people shouldn't exist in a modern country. We are constantly striving for progress, and it's just sad to see someone who is mentally challenged because even though they might not realize they are, everyone around them has to deal with them and the burden they put on others."

What many don't realize is the abortion movement in America didn't originate out of the women's movement or a right to privacy. It came from eugenics and served as a way to eradicate "human weeds." Those with mental disabilities were the first to be sterilized. The goal was to have people like this eradicated. Babies who had differences like this were aborted. Margaret Sanger, founder of Planned Parenthood, was a eugenicist instrumental in this field, so it is no surprise that eugenics is still the goal of the abortion movement today.

The reality is that all of these children who are described as "less wanted" are safer in the womb of a pro-life mom. The pro-life movement is the widest embrace of life. It affirms the preciousness of life across the board and I applaud all parents who raise kids, whether they have special needs or not, with the unconditional love they deserve. Liz Crowter, a mom to a child with Down syndrome, told Channel 5 News in the UK, "Bringing up a child with Down syndrome is very challenging and hard work but my other three children are challenging and hard work as well, that is parenting. Her siblings are her best advocates."

Frank Stephens, an international advocate for human rights, has Down syndrome and has lived with it his whole life. He told the United Nations in 2018: "I am a man. See me as a human being, not a birth defect, not a syndrome. I don't need to be eradicated."[309] He also said, "I need to be loved, valued, educated, and sometimes helped." He also spoke to the U.S. Senate in 2017. He told them: "I am a man with Down syndrome and my life is worth living."[310] These statements are heartbreaking for the audience because the fact that he has to plead to the rest of us that his life is worth living shows how lost our society is. He has more heart than many politicians these days. Should the fact that a baby in the womb has an extra chromosome be a death sentence? Of course not. I agree with Mike Huckabee, who says that a child with Down syndrome is "just as important as the captain of the football team."[311]

"What If the Baby Has a Terminal Illness and Is Going to Die Anyway, Maybe Right after Being Born?"

A good friend of mine brought up Tay-Sachs disease and asked, "How could you force a mother to give birth to a baby for it to die in her arms?" Tay-Sachs can range from mild to severe and is extremely rare but if found in an infant is typically more severe and can result in the death of the child at an early age. My friend said that if she were pregnant and if blood tests and a genomic panel were done on the child in the womb and it was found to have the disease, then she would have an abortion. She said she met a woman in this situation and thought her story was convincing. The child and the mother would be better off if the baby were dead because the journey seemed so emotionally trying for the parents. My friend argued that it would be selfish for the mother to kill the baby before it's born, but she could understand that reasoning.

Whenever someone brings up terminal patients, I think about this. The reality is we are all on death row. We are all going to die. We know this. We all live next to a ticking clock. Sometimes we think about this truth, and sometimes we don't. But whether or not we die is not up for debate. It's just a matter of when. What gives you the right to cut off this person's life early? If a baby dies of natural causes that is one thing, but they should not die at the hand of their mother or the state.

The goal of leftists is for these babies to die, but they have human dignity, a right to life, and should be loved and medically treated. Even if the child has a terminal illness, we shouldn't kill it simply because it is a person and persons have natural rights. It doesn't matter if the person is going to die in a week, a month, five years, or fifty years, that does not change their status of personhood or give us the right to kill them. To say that someone doesn't have a high quality of life and use it as an excuse to kill them is a very slippery slope. If the baby's death is so imminent, why do we have to be their executioner?

Some babies die at an early age due to something like a car accident. That doesn't mean their life was not worth anything. And to intentionally kill a child is completely different. Even if we could kill terminally ill children before birth, it would not make sense to do so because testing is not foolproof, meaning there is a chance you are killing a perfectly healthy person. Killing the child before it is born only allows the potential for a healthy baby to be killed unnecessarily.

Regarding Tay-Sachs specifically, there is medication to prevent seizures that is very effective as well as respiratory care. We should focus on finding cures to these diseases, not killing babies. Gene therapy and enzyme replacement therapy may eventually lead to a cure or stop the progression of that disease. One thing that is important to remember is that babies get heart transplants and can have brain surgery. Babies born without a rectum, uterus, or any other parts of that nature can have surgery as well. I don't see the argument here, since medical technology is so advanced and continues to improve.

My friend insisted that the emotional pain of the parents would be too much. I pointed out that many people experience emotional pain that's not a justification for killing a third party. In order to help the parents deal with a particularly emotionally trying situation, we should encourage support groups and increased resources to aid their mental health, so that parents know they are not alone. Support groups are immensely helpful to parents with a sick child as well as a sick spouse, parent, or friend. Various psychologists have also written powerful books on the subject as well as blogs, so helping parents through a situation like this is critical and the emotional pain they go through should not be ignored or diminished.

Most parents who have a child with them on Earth for only a week don't regret that week they spent together. Even women who have a miscarriage feel a sense of loss. And that's because it's life. It's a person, so we feel something for them. That's normal, and we should feel something. Addressing these emotions as opposed to killing the child is the solution here. I am not debating whether it is emotionally painful for the parents; this situation is incredibly painful. It's heart-wrenching, but loving the baby through its natural life and aborting the baby is something very different.

In sum, when we think about these hard cases, I ask you this: Do the 3 percent of abortions due to rape, incest, disability, or danger to life of the mother justify the death of the other 97 percent of babies aborted? Of course not.

BETTER OFF DEAD

"I have feelings too. I am still human." [312]

—MARILYN MONROE, *who grew up in foster care for a period of her childhood*

CHAPTER SEVENTEEN

MYTH: The fate of babies born alive as the result of a botched abortion is a decision between a woman and her doctor. Such complications are rare and do not diminish a woman's right to choose.

"Shoot straight you bastards, shoot! Don't make a mess of it."[313]

—HARRY MORANT, in the film *Breaker Morant*

What if an abortion is attempted and the child lives? This seems like an almost unthinkable situation, but it happens. Should we let it live? Should we kill it on the doctor's table? These are the hard cases that get far less attention from the Left. Just as cases of abortion due to incest and rape are extremely rare, children born from botched abortions are also rare. But that doesn't mean we shouldn't discuss them. Just as we should discuss cases of rape and incest, we should discuss botched abortions. This is the issue

Democrat governor Ralph Northam weighed in on with his controversial comments, even though he is still the governor of Virginia today.

Babies Killed Outside the Womb

But first, for some background, let's look back at some eye-opening testimony from the year 1999. In a hearing before U.S. Congress in Washington, DC, a nurse named Jill Stanek stood up and addressed Congress with this description:

> The method of abortion that Christ Hospital in Oaklawn, Illinois, uses is called "induced labor abortion," also now known as "live birth abortion." This type of abortion can be performed different ways, but the goal always is to cause a pregnant woman's cervix to open so that she will deliver a premature baby who dies during the birth process or soon afterward. The way that induced abortion is most often executed at my hospital is by the physician inserting a medication called Cytotec into the birth canal close to the cervix. Cytotec irritates the cervix and stimulates it to open. When this occurs, the small, pre-term baby drops out of the uterus, *oftentimes alive*. It is not uncommon for one of these live aborted babies to linger for an hour or two or even longer. One of them once lived for almost eight hours. In the event that a baby is aborted alive, he or she receives no medical assessments or care but is only given what my hospital calls "comfort care." "Comfort care" is defined as keeping the baby warm in a blanket until he or she dies, although even

this minimal compassion is not always provided. It is not required that these babies be held during their short lives.

Stanek related another personal experience:

One night, a nursing co-worker was taking an aborted Down's Syndrome [sic] baby who was born alive to our Soiled Utility Room because [the little boy's] parents did not want to hold him, and she did not have time to hold him. I could not bear the thought of this suffering child dying alone in a Soiled Utility Room, so I cradled and rocked him for the 45 minutes that he lived. He was 21 to 22 weeks old.... Toward the end he was so quiet that I couldn't tell if he was still alive unless I held him up to the light to see if his heart was still beating through his chest wall. After he was pronounced dead, we folded his little arms across his chest, wrapped him in a tiny shroud, and carried him to the hospital morgue where all of our dead patients are taken.

The nurse then offered another example: "A Support Associate told me about a live aborted baby who was left to die on the counter of the Soiled Utility Room wrapped in a disposable towel. This baby was accidentally thrown into the garbage, and when they later were going through the trash to find the baby, the baby fell out of the towel and on to the floor." She said, "We look the other way and pretend that these babies aren't human while they're alive but human only after they are dead. We issue these babies both birth and death certificates, but it is really only the death certificate that matters. No other children in America are medically abandoned like this."

Then, commenting on what she had just reported, Nurse Stanek added, "Abortion is a cancer that is literally killing America. It is killing our children while it is killing our consciences. It began when we took God out of our decision-making and proclaimed that the little beings growing inside of women were 'products of conception' and not little girls and little boys. Who should be surprised that we keep pushing the envelope so that now we are aborting these 'products of conception' alive?"[314]

This testimony exposed the extremes to which the pro-choice, or rather, pro-abortion movement was willing to go. *Roe* never contemplated late-term abortions or infanticide. The debate hadn't gone there yet. Nobody thought we were talking about this kind of circumstance. But since *Roe v. Wade*, the floodgates have opened and babies are being intentionally killed or left to die outside the womb. Jill Stanek's testimony was a pivotal turning point, calling out the horrors that have become part of our culture.

One would think that these instances are extremely rare. But they happen far too often. In 1997, Ron Fitzsimmons, executive director of the National Coalition of Abortion Providers, estimated that the method was used three thousand to five thousand times annually. "In the vast majority of cases, the procedure is performed on a healthy mother with a healthy fetus that is 20 weeks or more along," Fitzsimmons said.[315] In November 1995, Mr. Fitzsimmons recalled the night in when he appeared on *Nightline* on ABC and "lied through my teeth" when he said the procedure was used rarely and only on women whose lives were in danger or whose fetuses were damaged.[316] In January 2003, even the Guttmacher Institute—an affiliate of Planned Parenthood—published a survey of abortion providers that estimated that 2,200 abortions were performed by this method in the year 2000.[317]

The Born Alive Infant Protection Act (BAIPA) was signed into law by President George W. Bush in 2002 in order to prevent doctors from killing babies outside the womb, even if they had intended to abort them. It states: "the words 'person,' 'human being,' 'child,' and 'individual' shall include every infant member of the species *homo sapiens* who is born alive...at any stage of development."[318] One would think this would be a nonpartisan issue—one that both Republicans and Democrats would support. But this is not so.

The Democratic Party wants these babies killed. President Bill Clinton vetoed a bill that would have outlawed the controversial procedure in 1997. There were enough opponents in the House of Representatives to override his veto but not in the Senate. As an Illinois senator, Barack Obama voted against the Born Alive Infant Protection Act twice; as chairman of the Health and Human Services Committee in 2003, he prevented it from advancing to the floor. Obama then became a two-term president, and between 2008 and 2016 we saw the radicalization of the Democratic Party and the abortion debate. Now, the Democratic Party platform advocates for abortions when a woman is nine months pregnant. Where does it stop?

Governor Northam of Virginia is only the latest installment of the Democratic support of what amounts to infanticide. Northam supported born-alive abortions last year and used the explicit language of "comfort care." Northam, a pediatric neurosurgeon, said of an infant intended to be aborted, "The infant would be delivered. The infant would be kept comfortable. The infant would be resuscitated if that's what the mother and the family desired. And then a discussion would ensue between the physicians and the mother." He added, "We want the government not to be involved in these types of decisions. We want the decision to be made by the mothers and their providers."[319] He was not asked to step down by other Democrats in his party. Ralph Northam, whose nickname in college was "Coonman," was even caught having dressed up with a friend. One was dressed as a KKK member in a full hood and the other in blackface, and the Democrats still would not denounce Northam. The Democrats will stop at nothing to fulfill their pro-abortion agenda, and since Northam is one of them, they protect him.

This horror is seeping through our nation. There are babies to this day who are born alive and thrown in trash cans to die.[320] Nothing leads us to believe that these procedures are practiced less often today than in 1997. We can assume this because of the vehement opposition to the bill Republicans are trying to pass, which would hold people accountable for killing these children after they are born. Called the Born-Alive Abortion Survivors Protection Act, it is intended "to prohibit a health care practitioner from failing to exercise the proper degree of care in the case of a child who survives an abortion or attempted abortion." It shouldn't be controversial at all, but it is. Why would Democrats try to stop this if in fact infants were no longer born alive and killed? It is likely that they are covering for their abortion clinic counterparts, organizations like Planned Parenthood, whom they support and who conduct these atrocities.

Hippocratic Oath

The purpose of medicine is healing. It's to take people who are sick or dying and make them better. The irony of abortion is if an abortion is successful, you end up with a dead child. If the abortion fails, you end up with a live baby that you have just tried to kill, who is likely physically harmed from the experience. This is an inversion of the Hippocratic Oath. Doctors who take part in performing abortions other than to preserve the life of the mother are violating their ethic to save lives. Killing is killing. This may be lawful killing, but if you are not saving a life, you are purely killing.

Survivors of Abortion

There are millions of successful abortions—sixty-one million and counting in America since *Roe v. Wade*. And out of these abortions come dead bodies. There are also unsuccessful abortions, which are often called botched abortions. These are babies that abortionists tried to kill but something went wrong in the process and the baby somehow lived through it. Some of these children were killed outside the womb, as described above, by being left to die in a utility room with no nutrients. The general practice after a baby is born alive is to kill it by suffocation, strangulation, leaving the baby to die, or throwing the baby away. Many are thrown into trash cans, literally discarded. But depending on the particular abortion clinic, some of these survivors are sent to an emergency room where they are revived and treated, and some are alive today. Many of these survivors have physical deformities and other permanent scars from their horrific experience. Some are mentally handicapped—some more functional than others—but most are permanently scarred from the procedure.

Gianna Jessen is an abortion survivor. It says so on her medical records: "born during saline abortion." Her birth certificate was signed by her abortionist. A saline abortion is when saline is injected into the womb. The baby is poisoned and burned alive. It typically takes about an hour for the baby to die. A day or so later, the mother gives birth to a stillborn. Somehow, Gianna was born alive. "I should be blind, I should be burned, I should be dead," says Gianna. "But I'm not."[321] In Gianna's case, a nurse called an ambulance, and she was transferred to a hospital. She was placed in an emergency foster care home. Today she has cerebral palsy.

Her cerebral palsy was caused by the lack of oxygen to her brain when she was trying to survive in the womb while the abortionist was trying to kill her with saline. Before she was injected with saline, she was a perfectly healthy baby. She wouldn't have cerebral palsy had it not been for this direct attack on her. She lived in foster care until she was adopted at age four. One may wonder how a person like Gianna can go through life without anger. But she does say this: "If abortion were merely about women's rights, what were mine?"

But she is incredibly strong. "You didn't get me. The silent Holocaust didn't win over me," she says. She knows she has been hated since conception, but she also knows she is loved by the only one whose love matters, and that's God. "I'm His girl," she says.

Gianna is disgusted by arguments that say that women should have abortions because the child might be disabled. She speaks about how the Lord loves the weakest in society and what arrogance it is to argue that you are better than someone else. She has forgiven her biological mother. She has forgiven those who have hurt her. She is focused on the future and has dedicated her life to speaking up for the voiceless. She is hated by many on the Left because she represents what they hate, and that is hope for an end to abortion.

She represents the living consequence of what it means to harm another human being. She speaks out, and they don't like it.

Gianna is just one of many survivors of an abortion attempt. Another is Melissa Ohden, who, despite fears of terrible disabilities, grew up to live a perfectly healthy life with an adoptive family. But emotionally, she was crippled. She grew up and found her birth mother, who had no idea she had survived the abortion. It was a defining moment in Melissa's life to meet her mother. She learned that the abortionist who performed the procedure on her was a friend of her family. She forgave her birth mother and cultivated a relationship with her. Melissa changed and ended up being grateful for her life. She now says, "I am one of the luckiest people in the world."[322]

Another is Claire Culwell. Her birth mother had an abortion when she was five months pregnant. But little did she know she was pregnant with twins. One of the babies died, but the other survived. The baby that survived, Claire, was born with dislocated hips and club feet. Claire now says, "I was in body casts to correct what the abortion had done."[323] Another is Josiah Presley, who was maimed due to an attempt to kill him by the suction method of abortion. He survived. He was adopted and loved and says of preborn children, "They are innocent and can't defend themselves against these huge abortion bullies killing them."[324]

Stories like Gianna's and Josiah's are not typical, but neither are they uncommon. Chip Roy (R-TX) stood up among other congressmen in November 2019 and related the moving story of a child who underwent being aborted but lived through it. The doctors encouraged the parents to complete the abortion after it had failed, but the parents said to let the child and his twin live. He then said that one of those children was on the house floor and pointed to him. Sure enough, he is one of the staffers working for the congressman.[325] The room was left in awe.

How many more children will we let this happen to? These people were tortured and lived to tell the tale. While the Left tries to silence them, their voices are louder than ever and more inspiring than ever. We must fight for their lives and the lives of the unborn.

CHAPTER EIGHTEEN

MYTH: Research shows that the children who would have otherwise been aborted usually become criminals, wreaking havoc on all of us. It may be selfish, but we all want crime rates to drop, and abortion provides undeniable social benefits.

"The problem with pragmatism is that it doesn't work."

—G. K. CHESTERTON

Could it be that abortion produces important social benefits? Could it be that making abortion illegal would cause destructive social pathologies? Precisely such an argument has been made in favor of abortion. It was made by two scholars, Steven Levitt of the University of Chicago and John Donohue of Stanford University, in a paper that made quite a splash when it was published in 2001.

Levitt popularized the thesis in a best-selling book that he coau-thored with Stephen Dubner called *Freakonomics*. In fact, Levitt and Donohue's argument is so famous that it is sometimes referred to simply as "the Freakonomics argument."

The argument, in fact, focuses on crime. Crime rates in Amer-ica were very high in the 1970s, and they declined dramatically in the 1990s. Levitt and Donohue argue that one of the reasons—not the only reason, but one of the main reasons—for this decline was abortion, which increased drastically after *Roe v. Wade*. Quite sim-ply, they argued that abortion reduced the number of unwanted children in America, and these unwanted children, had they been born, were more likely to become criminals. The decline of crime, therefore, in their view, can be directly traced to the elimination of these unwanted prospective criminals from the population.

To quote Levitt and Donohue, "Abortion is an efficient way to curtail future crime. It's a simple math problem." Pro-abortion advocates have jumped on this argument, and they like it because it's an argument that appeals to safety. If you want to live in a soci-ety that's more orderly, that has less crime, one way to do that is to eliminate children whose unfortunate lives are more likely to push them in the direction of criminality. I must say that on the New York cocktail circuit this argument, among the "limousine liber-als," the classic rich Democrat, the Freakonomics argument is very popular.

Levitt and Donohue approach their argument with some cau-tion. They do say that their argument is not a reason to become an advocate for abortion. In fact, Levitt even says that if you believe that the fetus is the moral equivalent of a person, then the trade-off of trying to get lower crime rates by killing human beings is awful. It makes no sense. Levitt even says, "You are misguided if you use our study to base your opinion about what the right policy is toward abortion." These caveats notwithstanding, Levitt and Donohue do say that current efforts to regulate abortion such as heartbeat bills are making future crime rates more likely to go up, and so they have hung tough on their argument. To some degree it is understandable why pro-choice advocates have adopted this argument because it draws a direct connection between pro-choice laws, *Roe v. Wade* if you will, and the welcome decline of crime in America in the last few decades.

Since pro-abortion people, despite these caveats, embrace the idea, let's seriously consider the argument from *Freakonomics*. First of all, let's for a moment presume that the argument is completely true. Let's presume that abortion does have the social benefits just as Levitt and Donohue suggest. All that would seem to prove is that forms of oppression, even murderous forms of oppression, can sometimes have unintended positive consequences. There's a very interesting book written by the German historian Götz Aly called *Hitler's Beneficiaries*. Aly asks the question "Why did the Germans support Hitler to the very end?" His answer in part is that they did so because Hitler was a socialist. He had an expansive welfare state that provided all kinds of social benefits to the German people: retirement benefits, income supplements, unemployment insurance, health care, and so on.

But then Aly raises the question: How did Hitler fund all that? Where did he get the money? And the answer is very simple. He got the money by looting the Jews within Germany, and he got the money by looting captive peoples in Europe outside Germany. The German people enjoyed some of the benefits of him stealing and the benefit of his murderous rampage; it made life easier for people in Germany after World War I, and that's why the German people hung tough with Hitler. It wasn't that they all liked Hitler as a person or they agreed with Hitler or they even knew everything he was doing, but they actually derived benefits from his stolen goods. Here we see a way in which Hitler's terrible oppression and mass murder delivered a social benefit to the German people.[326]

Some argue that slavery, a terrible form of oppression, produced some economic and social benefits for the oppressors and others in the society at the time. One of its social benefits was to make dirt-poor white laborers and farmers in the South have higher self-esteem. These white laborers were at the very bottom of society, but thanks to slavery they could always say that their social status was higher than that of the slave, than that of the black man, and so slavery supplied a kind of psychological floor above which all white people were placed. However, I think no person in their right mind would condone this form of oppression on the basis that the enslaving of some produced the social benefit of raising the self-image of others.

In the case of Levitt and Donohue's argument, even if crime rates would become lower by aborting certain groups, that does not justify aborting people in low-income neighborhoods. In fact, let's push that thinking even further. Presumably, one could eliminate all crime produced by a particular cohort of young people by killing them all off before they were born. In other words, imagine an abortion rate of 100 percent. No children are born in that area at all. Obviously, if you then look twenty or twenty-five years later, you'll discover that that age group hasn't committed any crime. Why? Because they don't exist. When pushed to the extreme, the argument is exposed. The argument that the way to get less crime is to preemptively kill off all the potential people who could do those crimes is not an argument that holds up.

This notion that there are people in the world who are in some way predisposed to become criminals has its roots in a very real and sick ideology: eugenics. Eugenics is the idea that the quality of a population—be it the race, gender, intellectual, or moral quality—can be improved by selecting or getting rid of people who will pollute the community. These people will bring down the average national IQ, commit crimes, look ugly, and pull the country downward in some way. The eugenics argument was actually cited by Justice Clarence Thomas in May 2019 when the Supreme Court turned down an abortion-related appeal in Indiana. Referencing eugenics, Thomas specifically cited *Freakonomics* and linked its argument to Planned Parenthood founder Margaret Sanger, who was a dedicated champion of eugenics and well-known racist.[327]

I want to zoom into Levitt and Donohue's argument more closely to see whether the correlation it establishes between legal abortion and reduced crime rates actually holds up because this is the crux of their argument. While I clearly dispute the morality of eugenics, of killing people in certain groups for some perceived social benefit, it is clear that their argument isn't supported by real evidence.

In some places, specifically New York City, their argument appears to hold up—until you look more closely. There actually is a correlation in New York. Legal abortions went up, up, up in the 1970s after *Roe v. Wade* in 1973, and in New York crime went down, down, down in the late 1980s and 1990s. So naturally, New York is an example they might look at to support their argument. But this pattern doesn't hold for other cities. If you look at Newark, right across from New York City, or look to Baltimore, a couple of hundred miles south of New York, we find that abortion went up in the 1970s, but crime was also up. In fact, the rate of violence in Baltimore is climbing faster than ever before. The level of violence in Baltimore is the highest it's ever been to this day.[328] And the level of violence remains high in Newark as well. So, while New York and Newark looked similar twenty-five or thirty years ago, now their crime rates are quite different. Cincinnati also hasn't seen a sharp decline in violence. So, what this means is that it's more likely that policies specific to New York City produced the decline of the New York crime rate and not the common thread of abortions, which had been going up through the 1970s and 1980s in all of these cities.

So, then, why did crime actually go down? It's very easy to see why that happened, particularly in New York. Crime rates went down because mayors like Rudy Giuliani began to adopt a get-tough policy on crime. Quite simply, the authorities began to lock up the criminals, take them off the street—and this, by the way, doesn't apply only to serious criminals, like murderers and rapists. The focus was also on petty criminals, like burglars. Studies showed that petty criminals often graduate to more serious forms of crime, and moreover they create an atmosphere in which crime becomes more acceptable and people live in fear.

This is known as "the broken windows theory." The idea is that if you walk into a poor neighborhood and you see a broken window and you come back a week later and that broken window is not fixed, it is very likely that in subsequent weeks more windows will be broken in that neighborhood. Why? Because the unfixed window sends the message to the community, "Nobody cares about these things. Property rights are ultimately not being protected in this neighborhood. The cops are powerless. Break-ins cannot be stopped. You can break windows with impunity"; and so it happens. There was a real crackdown on crime in the 1980s and 1990s; Americans got sick of crime. In places like New York there were very effective policies put into place. That's the overwhelming reason why crime rates went down. Abortion had little if anything to do with it.

I think the authors of *Freakonomics* have preposterously exaggerated the risk of a child becoming a criminal. Let's consider a poor woman in a poor area of the country who is pregnant. She decides to carry the baby to term and not get an abortion, and let's say this is in 1974, right after *Roe v. Wade* passed and before crime was cleaned up wherever she lives. First of all, the woman has a fifty-fifty chance of having a girl or a boy. If she has a girl, what's the chance that that girl is going to become a violent criminal? Statistically, very low. The vast majority of violent crimes are committed by males. Right away we eliminate 50 percent of the chance that we're going to have a violent criminal on our hands.

The second issue is, if the woman has the baby, she has two choices. She can keep the baby and raise it in her neighborhood, which is perhaps a dysfunctional environment, or she can give the child up for adoption. If the child is given up for adoption, suddenly the unwanted child becomes a wanted child. It might not have been wanted by her, but it's wanted by another couple who decides to raise it. What is the chance that this adoptive child placed in a wanted home will now become a criminal? Much lower. In fact, it is Levitt and Donohue's own argument that "unwantedness" is a decisive factor that leads to criminality. The point here is that Levitt and Donohue have grossly exaggerated the chances that unwanted children born post-*Roe* in cities will become violent criminals.

In closing this argument, there's something particularly strange and repulsive about killing people before they have done anything wrong. Should someone be killed based solely on the idea that he or she might do something wrong? At the end of the day, that's what the Levitt and Donohue argument comes to.

To assume that someone will become a criminal, to assume that they are nothing more than a statistic, sets them up for failure. There are so many rich Democrats who think like this, and it can become a self-fulfilling prophesy for others because this ideology seeps into the culture. So many people in inner cities have a sense of despair and hopelessness because their Democrat leaders, who have been their leaders for decades, don't think enough of them to actually create any opportunities. Instead, they want them to remain dependent on the government. Many Democrats don't think it's worth it to change the inner-city environments in which people grow up. They just want to put a bandage on the problem— often in the form of handouts from the government.

Anyone may become a criminal, but there are so many success stories. When you kill off a population of people, you lose all the bad things that they might do, but you also lose all the good things that they might do. There might be an Einstein in the group. There might be a Picasso. There might be people who don't achieve extraordinary things but still live decent, lawful, meaningful lives. Those lives are lost because we kill off those people; we as a society decide it's okay to kill off those people on the chance that some of them might go down the wrong road. Who is one of the most intelligent minds you can think of? What is one of the items you probably can't live without? Steve Jobs, inventor of the iPhone, could have been aborted.

Steve Jobs's mother could have chosen to get an illegal abortion but instead chose to give him up for adoption. She was Catholic, so adoption was encouraged, and she went to a shelter for unwed mothers that delivered babies and found homes for them. Steve Jobs said in an interview, "I wanted to meet my biological mother mostly to see if she was okay and to thank her because I'm glad I didn't end up as an abortion. She was twenty-three and went through a lot to have me."[329]

If Steve Jobs was one in a million, and sixty-one million babies have been aborted in America since *Roe v. Wade*, what does that mean for our country? It means that we are missing out on geniuses like him, and we will never know the amazing things those people could have accomplished. Even if we account for some of them not being productive members of society or just being consumers and takers rather than contributing, the benefits of the minds of a few like Jobs would have provided immense benefits to millions of people. President Trump said, "We cannot know what our citizens yet unborn will achieve, the dreams they will imagine."[330] This is true. If they are not born and are killed in the womb, we will never know.

Is it bad to be born in an environment riddled with crime, violence, gangs, drugs, broken homes? Of course. It's terrible. We need to improve the educational opportunities of children who grow up in difficult neighborhoods. We need to be tough on crime so families are safe. It's not just poverty but the lack of a father figure that leads many young males to join gangs, seeking a community and family there. What underpins any society is the family.

In order to restore the family structure in America, as well as in inner-city neighborhoods, we must begin by stopping abortion. Abortion may seem like a "quick fix" but only results in spreading despair and a culture of death in that community. Abortion devalues human life. Fostering a culture of cherishing human life is the first step in stopping the vicious cycle of violence in communities.

CHAPTER NINETEEN

MYTH: Unwanted children will be a burden on the welfare state. Unless you're personally going to provide for them, you can shut up. Pro-life people profess to care so much about the child before it's born, but then after it's born, they don't want to pay for it.

"It is a poverty that a child must die, so that you may live as you wish."[331]

—MOTHER TERESA, Calcutta

Pro-choicers respond to pro-lifers by saying something like this: How can the country be expected to support all of these unwanted children if you make abortion illegal? You're going to have a huge spike in the number of unwanted children, born to poor, dysfunctional families on welfare. This creates a massive burden that we all have to bear. A burden on the welfare state. It becomes a burden on society in general. Do you have any plans for providing for these people? Comedian George Carlin says, "Boy, these conservatives are really something, aren't they? They're all in favor of the unborn. They will do anything for the unborn. But once you're born, you're on your own. Pro-life conservatives are obsessed with the fetus from conception to nine months. After that, they don't want to know about you. They don't want to hear from you."[332]

The argument continues: You pro-lifers profess to care so much about the child before it's born. But after it's born, you disclaim all responsibility. You want a population explosion, but you don't want to pay for it. You don't want to provide the kinds of services, educational services, health care services, and so on, that are necessary for people to live full lives; so goes the claim of the pro-choice advocates.

Here's my reply: First of all, the claim is based on the assumption that population growth is a serious problem in the United States, perhaps in other industrialized countries as well. And this is a refrain that we've heard now for many years. In fact, it goes back a couple of hundred years to Thomas Malthus, father of the dire Malthusian prophecy. He claimed that resources grow arithmetically, which is to say 1, 2, 3, 4, 5, or gradually; but populations grow, he said geometrically, 2, 4, 6, 8, and so on. And if you do the math, Malthus said you can see very quickly that population will outstrip available resources and countries will become impoverished. Malthus's theory has been about as well refuted as any sociological theory in history.

By and large, we've seen swelling populations in all the developed countries. Far from being accompanied by impoverishment, this population growth has been accompanied by rising living standards virtually through every generation, perhaps not counting the two world wars. The Cato Institute has studied this question in detail, and its studies have shown that America's growing population has actually been critical to establishing America as an economic superpower, indeed a world superpower.

Now, how is this possible? How can it be that more people make a country economically stronger as well as stronger in other ways? Well, the answer is really simple. People in general are an economic asset. Yes, people consume: they consume food, they consume space, and so on, but people also *produce*. And if you look at human beings over a lifetime, their productive capacities on average and in general outweigh what they take from society. They put more into the pot, you might say, than they take out.

Countries that are developed today, far from having a problem of too many people, have a problem of too few people. On average, it takes a little over two children for a couple to reproduce itself. The reason it's a little more than two is because of mortality, accidents, and so on. So by and large, you have to have two kids or more to keep society just where it is. And the problem is that the average American couple today does not have even two kids, so America's population under normal circumstances would be shrinking. This is also the case for Europe, Japan, and other countries. They are facing the prospect of shrinking populations because they are not reproducing to replace themselves. In America's case, our population increases due to immigration. It is the influx of immigrants from the outside that has kept America's population growing at a fairly modest pace, but were it not for that, American population would be shrinking too.

Let's turn to the issue of immigration and specifically focus for a moment on illegal immigration. Strangely, the people who make the argument that the welfare state can't support unwanted children or can't support children who would otherwise be aborted are the same people who say, "Oh, yes, we can sustain illegal immigration. We can move toward something resembling open borders." In other words, they're willing to give all these same welfare state benefits to illegals, but not to the children of fellow Americans.

But wait a minute. If anyone is entitled to these benefits, shouldn't it be Americans? There are more than twenty-two million illegal immigrants living in the United States, according to a recent Yale study, which examined immigration rates between the years 1990 and 2016.[333] Since *Roe v. Wade* in 1973, over sixty-one million abortions have occurred in America.[334] So, if we had let all those children be born and did not have illegal immigrants, we could have easily taken care of about one-third of those children with the same welfare supports that are already allocated, with the same educational supports that are currently being used to support illegals, who are not paying taxes. The welfare state does not owe anything to people who are not citizens. The people who pay into it are citizens, so it should go to citizens. We also take in about a million legal immigrants, so illegal immigrants are basically skipping the line before all others also wanting to come legally. My own father is an immigrant who came here legally and had to wait about ten years before becoming a naturalized citizen.

When pro-choicers talk about the fear of increasing the burden on the welfare state, it's kind of funny because they don't seem to complain when the welfare state expands in other areas. In fact, they are the ones pushing to expand the welfare state. They are happy to see more people getting unemployment benefits. More people on food stamps? Great. Free health care for illegals? No problem. But when it comes to raising the children who would otherwise be aborted, the Left will suddenly balk at the prospect of this and claim the welfare state can't possibly handle that.

It is also important to note that the welfare state that leftists claim can't take on additional responsibilities is an irresponsible welfare state that the Left itself has created. Let's remember that the welfare state is not what it was intended to be. It has morphed into something else. The welfare state actually was intended to be a safety net, by and large for transitory or even emergency situations. Franklin Roosevelt justified federal programs in terms of supporting widows and orphans. Why? Because they are the most vulnerable citizens. At that time, destitute widows whose husbands were killed in war and their dependent children were also the concern of the state. The state was not intended to support able-bodied people who should work. But it seems perfectly logical that it should assist the most vulnerable in our society—the unborn.

If we had a responsible welfare state, none of the complaints about taking care of destitute babies would be necessary, and the issue of children potentially needing to be supported wouldn't be a problem either. Why? Because not every baby born would be on welfare. Babies born to people who are destitute also get adopted into homes that can afford to care for them. Babies also grow up and become contributors themselves. After all, they are not babies forever.

Allowing abortion on demand, far from diminishing the irresponsibility of the welfare state's culture, actually encourages it. Abortion sends the message: abort away, please do. The Left sends the message: we've set up Planned Parenthood locations right in your neighborhood, actually, mostly black neighborhoods, so go for that abortion. The welfare state says: but hey, if you do have a child and are on welfare, no worries, we'll give you more money.

This is a horrible system. We need to create a culture of personal responsibility where people are inclined to be responsible for their own actions as well as their own family. It is often fathers who step out of the picture, not providing for their children with a woman they do not live with. This needs to stop, and the answer to this isn't a further corruption of the family. When it comes to the welfare state, people should only be dependent on it if they are so helpless, so disabled, that they are not in a position to take care of themselves.

We've been focusing on dependency and on the welfare state, but not all babies who have been aborted since *Roe v. Wade* would have been on welfare. It isn't just people on welfare who get abortions. The argument that unwanted children become a burden on society is all based on the stereotype of poor children raised in the barrio or in the ghetto, poor children who are not going to be in a position to sustain themselves. And yet we need to remember that there are a large number of abortions by educated women, middle-class women, upper-middle-class women, successful women. These are not women on welfare, and these are not women who, if they had the child, wouldn't be able to care for it and send it to school.

Now, what about this notion that pro-lifers are hypocrites because they support saving the lives of the unborn and then don't care about the fate of the child after it is born? This accusation is not grounded in reality because pro-life and pro-family organizations and charities, including churches, do more for children than anyone else. It is not true that pro-life organizations don't care about children after they're born. In fact, a lot of pro-life organizations have programs to help new mothers transition into motherhood.

There are many crisis pregnancy centers that do great work. Consider for example the Metroplex Women's Clinics in Texas, which, in addition to providing pregnancy counseling and prenatal care like ultrasounds, also offer postnatal services, providing tangible things like baby clothes as well as job references for the mother and early health care. They also help women explore alternatives to abortion, like adoption.[335] There are other organizations that aid these pregnancy centers. The Vitae Foundation, for example, works with over 130 crisis pregnancy centers across the country and helps women find out about these centers so that they know where they can go to get the help they need.[336]

Motherhood is in fact a challenge, especially for single mothers. Pro-lifers understand this and help women to make that transition. Planned Parenthood, though the organization's name includes the word "parenthood," does not actually provide anything to women to help them be a parent. It can offer you a lot if you want an abortion, but if you are having a baby, what does it offer you? Absolutely nothing.

Aside from this, it isn't reasonable to fault pro-life organizations for not being able to take on the child-rearing of every child after birth. Consider the abolitionists who fought to end slavery. Their emphasis, correctly, was on one thing: ending slavery. They doubtlessly realized that once the slave was freed, that wouldn't solve the slave's problems. The slave might be uneducated, the slave might be unemployed, the slave might face unbearable racial prejudice. And many abolitionists took in slaves themselves. Many started schools. Many taught them skills so they could have jobs.

But imagine saying to an abolitionist, "You are a hypocrite. You claim to be against slavery, but once the slave is freed, are you going to give every slave a job? Are you going to pay for everything? What about housing? You're against slavery while the slave is a slave, but afterward you don't want to take on all the burdens of freedmen."

This accusation makes no sense at all because abolitionists were clearly fighting for another man's freedom. In the case of abortion, the leftists arguing that pro-life people must bear the burden of child-rearing is saying this only to argue that the child should be dead. What they won't face is that improving someone's quality of life is impossible if they are dead.

CHAPTER TWENTY

MYTH: Unwanted children are better off not being born into this world. Children born into extreme poverty, homes of sexual abuse, and situations of suffering should not be forced to go through that. They are better off dead.

"I feel fine, considering the alternative."[337]

—RONALD REAGAN, when asked how he felt about turning seventy-nine

"Every child should be a wanted child." This is one of the slogans of the pro-choice movement. And behind it is a strong argument for the legality of abortion. The argument goes like this: lots of children live unwanted, miserable lives. If their parents don't want them, why bring them into the world? Many children who are aborted come from broken homes, areas with gang violence. They are conceived out of wedlock. They have parents on drugs. They clearly would live miserable lives. There's very little hope for them and those environments. They really are better off dead.

People who work in the foster care system have pointed out that they see very young children who are mistreated, sexually abused, burned with cigarettes, and subjected to painful, horrible conditions. Some of them come to believe that these children don't have a life worth living. They would be better off if they were prevented from coming into the world and experiencing so much pain. So why torture them by bringing them into this world?

I agree that being unwanted is a very bad situation for any child. After all, children are dependent on their parents, completely dependent in the very early years and largely dependent for many years after that. And if your parent or parents don't want you, then the chances are that they will not take care of you very well or that they will neglect you and treat you the way people treat something that they don't want.

The argument about unwantedness, and the idea that a child is being set up to have a painful life, rests on a hidden premise. And that premise is that pain and pleasure are the two governing principles of life. If pain is going to outweigh pleasure, or if one is being set up for a life largely made up of pain, that life is then not worth living. The thinking is that our purpose in life is to maximize pleasure and minimize pain. And if pain is really in your future, you're better off not existing at all. This argument was first made, I believe, by the philosopher Epicurus, and it is sometimes called the Epicurean position. The modern name for it is a limited form of hedonism where pain versus pleasure is measured.

Let's evaluate this argument. Historically, of course, the distinction between the wanted child and the unwanted child would seem to be inapplicable. Historically, most pregnancies were unplanned. Children typically were conceived accidentally. In this respect, they were unwanted in the beginning. Being a parent is scary, and even a married couple may not be quite ready to have a child. They know intuitively it's going to completely change their life, and yet the actual experiences of history is that children become wanted once they are around. Imagine all the people today who have kids that they didn't want, didn't plan for when they had them. How many of those people today would genuinely say or feel, "Hey, I wish I didn't have my kid. I really wish I had aborted him or her." That is rare. It is profoundly abnormal.

Most parents who initially didn't want their kids later say, "Hey, I never could have imagined my life would have turned out like this. I never thought I could love someone so much." Or something like, "Yes, my kid has completely changed my world. And it has also changed me for the better. I can't imagine my life now without them."

Even in the extreme situation, just because someone is unwanted by a parent doesn't mean that they are unwanted by everyone. I think for example of the inner cities, where a lot of times when a single mother has a child and either doesn't want the child or is in no position to raise a child, but there's somebody else who does. The grandparents often step in. They're willing to take on the role of the parent. And of course, in other cases if the parent doesn't want the child, they can put the child up for adoption.

But now I want to face the pro-choice argument at its strong point and look at children who are abused and ask, "Are these children really better off dead?" Among kids I've spoken to who have grown up in foster care or in broken homes, I have yet to meet one who says that he wishes he had been aborted. A good friend of mine, Terrence Williams, is a comedian who was raised in terrible conditions. His mother was a drug addict. He was raised in a series of foster homes. He faced abuse there. But Terrence has a strong spirit. He has become successful; he's made the most of his life. I'm not saying that every child will reach Terrence's level of success or achieve his strength of spirit, but what I am saying is that they, like Terrence, all believe that they are better off alive. They would rather cling to life, even a difficult life and struggle, rather than simply throw in the towel and quit. They do not believe that they would be better off dead.

Consider all the children in Africa, in India, in poor parts of the world who have so little, with no one to care for them. These children often don't even have enough food, water, or medicine, let alone a caring environment. And yet they struggle, they survive, they even smile. Americans are always struck by the smiles they see on the faces of children in Africa and India, and it's because sometimes Americans are shocked to see that even poor, sick children find meaning in life. They experience the full range of human emotions, happiness as well as sadness.

Interestingly, the actor Jack Nicholson was born out of a pretty difficult situation. He didn't find this out until he was thirty-seven years old, when a reporter for *Time* magazine dug deep into his past while putting together a cover story on him. The woman Nicholson had always thought was his sister, June, was actually his mother. And the woman he always thought was his mother, Ethel, was actually his grandmother. Both were dead when Nicholson found out, so he called up his brother-in-law Shorty (who was actually his uncle). Shorty denied the questions from Nicholson but then gave the phone to his wife, Lorraine, who said that what he'd found out was true.

Jack Nicholson told *Rolling Stone* in the 1980s, "I don't have to question the abortion issue in my mind. It's an open-and-shut case where I'm concerned. As an illegitimate child born in 1937, during the Depression, to a broken lower-middle-class family, you are a candidate for—you're an automatic abortion with most people today."[338] Jack Nicholson describes himself as personally pro-life because of his experience. "I'm positively against it," he has said. "I don't have the right to any other view. If June and Ethel had been of less character, I never would have gotten to live. These women gave me the gift of life."[339] He describes his only emotion as one of gratitude, literally for his life.

Celine Dion is another celebrity who was almost aborted. Her mother had already had thirteen children, making her pregnancy with Celine number fourteen. Celine's mother was devastated that she was pregnant and wanted an abortion. She sought the advice of her priest, who encouraged her to have the child. Celine Dion told the *National Post*, "Once my mother got over her disappointment that an abortion was out of the question, she loved me as passionately as she'd love the last little ones."[340] Celine is pro-life because of this.

Justin Bieber's mother, Mallette, was a victim of sex abuse. She was two years old when her alcoholic father walked out the door and three years old when she was sexually molested by an array of family friends and other male visitors. She was "sexually violated so many times that it began to feel normal."[341] She came to view herself as "a dirty girl" and turned to drug addiction to numb her pain. She attributes much of her pain to the "void of having a father in my heart." She left home at sixteen and turned to petty crime and dealing in pot to pay for drugs. She had an on-again, off-again relationship with Justin Bieber's father, Jeremy Bieber, for about four years starting when she was fifteen. At seventeen she threw herself in front of a truck. She survived and was sent to a mental ward. This is where she first found Jesus, though she quickly returned to drugs when released and got back with Jeremy. Then she found out she was pregnant.

Everyone in her life told her to just get an abortion, but she says, "I knew that I had to do what it took. I just couldn't abort him." She was eighteen years old and living in a home for pregnant girls when Justin was born. She went on government assistance, and a neighbor paid for a year of Justin Bieber's day care. Mallette went back to school and earned her degree, vowing at age twenty-one not to have sex outside marriage and to follow her Christian faith. Justin started singing at age six, and the rest is history. Mallette revealed her story in her book *Nowhere but Up*. Justin Bieber has had his own share of drug issues, and this led him and his mom to become estranged. She never wanted that for him. Justin says, "I was distant because I was ashamed."[342] They were seen going to Hillsong church together in 2018. I pray that their future is nowhere but up.

Isn't nowhere but up what we should want for all children? I am not saying that all children will become celebrities, but I am saying that there is hope and that we should take chances on kids. It is not their fault that they are born into a tough situation, and we should do everything we can to improve their situation. If you genuinely feel that their lives are so miserable, literally unbearable, then you should do something to help them.

Should we just kill everyone who has a difficult upbringing? Both my parents were brought up in difficult environments, whether it's impoverished India in the case of my dad or the white working class in the case of my mom. My grandparents were brought up in even more difficult environments. My grandmother was a refugee during World War II who had to flee Burma with her family, leaving behind all of their possessions, and resettle in Bombay. My other grandmother in America lost her father at sixteen, worked in a factory, was injured, and lost her brother in the wake of World War II. Both have passed away in the last year, and I am sure they would not like to hear these "better off dead" arguments if they were alive. No child is better off dead.

What the most privileged in society often forget is that people rise up out of situations, as they have for all of history. The solution is not to kill people in bad environments, claiming you're doing them a favor. We should instead focus on bettering those environments. We should create a culture of wantedness. We also need to inspire people to have personal responsibility and to make good choices with what they do have in order to make a better life for themselves.

I can't imagine a more difficult environment than being born a slave. In the case of slavery, there were parents who wanted a child but the slaves always knew that they wouldn't have any control over the child's life or would have very little; literally, the child belonged to, was the property of, the master. And the master was going to use the child for its whole life to serve the economic needs of the master. So, what kind of a life would that be? Nevertheless, slaves had children. They did not believe that these children would be better off dead. And some of them made great lives for themselves. I think, for example, of Booker T. Washington, born a slave, and yet he went on to found the Tuskegee Institute and became one of the leading African Americans in the United States—an inspiration to this day to people around the world.

Mother Teresa, a pro-life nun, said of abortion, "Give that child to me. I want it. I will care for it. I am willing to accept any child who would be aborted and to give that child to a married couple who will love the child and be loved by the child." And I think what Mother Teresa was getting at here is that a child may be unloved by a parent but that child is not unloved by her, Mother Teresa, and it's not unloved by God. And as it grows up, it will take charge of its own life and become an individual who is not at the mercy of its parents or caretaker. Saying a child is unwanted does not make it any less human at birth. Life is the right of every person. Our worth as human beings should not be determined solely by whether our parents want us. That doesn't define worth at all. Human life has an intrinsic dignity, an intrinsic preciousness, an intrinsic worth. And it is that worth that determines our right to live.

CHAPTER TWENTY-ONE

MYTH: Bad things happen to a lot of people, and the aborted fetus is simply the victim of bad luck.

"Whenever I hear anyone arguing over slavery, I feel a strong impulse to see it tried on him personally."

—ABRAHAM LINCOLN, speech to Fourteenth Indiana Regiment, March 17, 1865[343]

One of the strongest arguments for abortion is the argument that since there are so many problems in the world and so many people suffering, then why focus on this? Why value these lives when there are so many other lives to value? It all comes down to luck. If you're born into a life that ends sooner rather than later, then join the club. Being aborted is your bad luck. It's the ideology that says, "Hey fetus, it sucks for you. Life is hard, and there are tons of people around the world who have a bad shake in life. There are people in Africa who go without water. There are people who die every day from malnutrition or disease, and so you, the unborn, have been dealt an unfortunate hand. You got a bad set of cards, and so you have to die. Your situation is no different from anyone else's who is suffering. You're not the first. It happens." This is a strange argument because we never hear it unless someone is speaking to us quietly and in confidence.

No one makes this kind of argument publicly. The argument is ultimately a private justification for abortion. A lot of the public arguments for abortion aren't really justifications. They're rationalizations. A rationalization is a way of supporting something that you believe anyway. You've already come to a conclusion, and you're going to give a reason, any kind of reason, to support it. But it's not necessarily the real reason you believe what you believe. A justification is why you actually hold a particular position, and with abortion it's clear that we have two types of arguments: public arguments that are mainly rationalizations and private arguments, what people really think, which are justifications. So, this falls into the category of what people really think, a justification. It's an unspoken argument, but people don't like to say it because it sounds really harsh. People will say things like this if they are in familiar company, but the fact that they don't say it openly doesn't mean they don't believe it.

This argument is ultimately based on a certain kind of realpolitik. We all get dealt a certain hand in life, and this is fair in a sense because the wheel of fortune is spun for all of us before we enter the world and it determines our fate. You can be born a rich person. You can be born a poor person. You can be born with a low IQ. You could be born with a high IQ. You can be born with a susceptibility to baldness. And that's just the way it is. That is, you may say, the natural order of things, and we have no alternative but to accept it.

There are people who pretend to care about things. They pretend to be deeply upset about the injustices in the world. They pretend to be deeply moved by the plight of the Thai factory worker or the illegal alien or even the snail darter. These are fashionable causes. People pretend to care about them because it makes them look good to their friends without their having to sacrifice anything. (Very few actually stop riding on planes in protest of climate change, and very few stop buying clothes made in factories.) But they're not going to even pretend to care about a fetus because it doesn't help them in any way. This is not a fashionable cause, at least not in contemporary, left-wing culture. Professing your concern for the unborn doesn't win you brownie points, and so there's no reason to pretend.

The appeal to luck and to the cards dealt by nature is ultimately an appeal to human selfishness. It rests on the underlying belief that we don't actually care about people who are in other situations, and we don't need to care. Our indifference to other people is actually correct. It is an advocacy, one may say, of selfishness, and the strength of the argument is that human nature is selfish.

Adam Smith, the great philosopher of capitalism, gives the example of sitting at your breakfast table, let's say, somewhere in America or in London, and you hear that there has been a terrible earthquake in China; thousands of people have been killed. What is your reaction? Smith says that your initial reaction is to feel terrible and to make some declamations about how unfortunate and tragic it is, but within a few minutes, he insists, you're right back to eating your breakfast. You essentially are in the same mood that you were before you found out about the earthquake. In other words, the earthquake doesn't affect you at all. Your selfishness is so consuming; in fact, to go further one might say that if you had an itch under your foot, that would bother you more than the prospect of thousands of people being wiped out in a natural calamity in some remote part of the world, and Adam Smith uses this example to say that our thinking about the world begins and is rooted in our own interests, our own welfare. Then we begin to care about others only reluctantly, only in lesser degrees, and one may say in concentric circles stretching out from ourselves and then reaching to first our family and then our neighbors and then maybe our larger community or country and only then, and in the slightest way, the rest of humanity.

Now, taking Adam Smith's argument on its face, we have an added puzzle with the abortion issue where we don't just have a mother watching with indifference as a child dies, we have a mother actively taking steps to kill her own child, and so selfishness normally includes the interests of our children and our family. This goes against what would seem to be the natural order. Normally, parents go out of their way to look out for their children. This is the cord of nature itself, and typically we interpret our own welfare, our own interests, as including the interests of our spouses and our children. And so we have to understand why the cord of nature gets broken in the case of abortion, in which the interest of the mother is seen as set against the interest of the child.

Selfishness has never been understood to be a virtue in two thousand years of Western civilization. The philosopher Ayn Rand is almost unique in the argument she makes in her book *The Virtue of Selfishness*. Rand argues that selfishness is good. She argues that the two-thousand-year tradition of condemning selfishness is wrong. After all, Rand says, we come into the world by ourselves. We struggle to survive and to flourish, and this is not only what we do but what, in Rand's view, we ought to do. Therefore, she says altruism is a kind of attack on human self-esteem. People have every right to think about themselves first and perhaps even last and to pay less attention to the wants and needs of others. In other words, we value them only to the degree that they help us.

One could say that even one's children, for example, become ultimately assets to their parents—and that the parents care about them but only because the children are seen as extensions of themselves. So, the parents in that case are still looking out for their self-interest. Where their self-interest contradicts the interests of others, Rand sides with the self. Rand says famously, "I swear by life and my love of it, that I will never live for the sake of another man, nor ask another man to live for mine."[344]

While Rand acknowledges the selfish side of human nature, there is also a side to human nature that is empathetic. Adam Smith, himself, understood this in a book that he wrote before *The Wealth of Nations*, a book called *The Theory of Moral Sentiments*. Adam Smith talked about the other side of human nature, and this is, you may say, the unselfish side, the empathetic side. Adam Smith argued that this, too, is basic to human beings. When we see somebody else in pain, someone who, for example, banged into a table and is buckled over, we cringe. Why? Because we know what it's like, what it feels like to bang into a table. We have banged into tables ourselves. We have felt the sharp pain, and so even though we're not feeling it now, we identify with others, and we feel for them. This is empathy, and empathy, Adam Smith argues, is what connects us to our fellow man. This empathy is not a repudiation of selfishness. In fact, it builds upon selfishness. We only know what it feels like for somebody else to feel pain because we have felt pain ourselves. Perhaps not the same pain, but we can relate to pain in our human experience.

I think here of the Golden Rule stated by Jesus in Matthew 7:12, "Do unto others as you would have them do unto you." This is in some ways understood as an appeal to altruism, to helping others, but notice that it helps others according to a standard dictated by selfishness itself. "Do unto others as you would have them do unto you" is based on the idea of how would you like to be treated. And that supplies the standard. Morality, far from denying selfishness, acknowledges it because we can put ourselves in the shoes of another.

Something that most human beings care about is the idea of justice. Justice in terms of just deserts, or rather, fairness. I want to focus here on John Rawls, the great philosopher of social justice in the twentieth century. Rawls offered a unique way to think about justice in his book *A Theory of Justice*, and I want to interpret the argument in its broadest sense. Before diving into his theory of justice, I would like to point out that Rawls himself was personally pro-choice.[345] In a lecture he gave at the University of Chicago, he attributes a majority of the pro-life argument to the religious domain.[346] I will be focusing here on the theory he is most famous for, which is his theory of justice.

Rawls begins by considering luck. We sometimes contrast luck with merit. We contrast, for example, something that happened accidentally, let's say, winning the lottery, with something that is achieved, such as working hard and getting high grades in a class. But Rawls says, "What a minute? How did you get those high grades? You were born with a high IQ or you had a favorable social environment when you were young, and this helped you develop study habits and the work ethic."

He believes that much of our position in life is due to luck. In fact, Rawls says virtually all of it is: from the position into which we were born, our family, even our DNA and IQ, which allow us to change the position we were born into. Rawls would say that the work ethic you learned was from modeling someone else. So, in other words, what Rawls is saying is that even things that are normally attributed to merit are in some sense the product of luck. And what is the moral status of luck? Rawls says that luck, by itself, is neither just nor unjust. Luck is just luck, but what we do with luck, what we as a society or what we as individuals do with a situation, is what determines whether we are acting justly or unjustly.

Whenever we try to establish a formula for a just society, Rawls says, we are very likely to create a society that benefits us. If you're an intellectual, you're going to say intellectuals should design society. If you're a banker, you may say bankers should run society. So, we have to create a thought experiment, where we don't know what position we'll be in, what job we'll be in in society, in order to think about what justice means.

He asks us to imagine the society that we are designing is as fair as possible. A society in which our own position in life is unknown. In other words, we begin by drawing the blueprint for the society. It can be an equal society, it could be an unequal society, but the society is set up in such a way that our luck of the draw is not known in advance. We don't know if we're going to be born a king or a peasant. We are under what he calls a "veil of ignorance."[347] We don't know if we're born a poor kid in the inner city or Bill Gates. In fact, to apply Rawls's experiment to our situation, we don't know if we'll be born at all. We don't know if we'll be aborted in the womb or left on the hillside to freeze to death, as was a common practice for the Spartans. We don't know. So, we have to design a society recognizing that we could end up in any of those positions. Now what kind of society, Rawls asks, would we design?

His answer is simple: we would design a society in which our prospects for a terrible outcome would be minimized. This makes sense. We wouldn't try to set up a society in which there is a reasonable chance that we would be killed or prevented from exercising our life choices. We would try to set up society in such a way that although there may be inequality and although some may have more than others, people have what the Declaration of Independence stated: "life, liberty, and the pursuit of happiness." We would also want to create a society with freedom and opportunity so that people had the chance to move up. We would want people to be protected from crime.

But even before we discuss how society would look as far as opportunity, merit, success, and all of the things life entails, we would try to design a society in which there is life in the first place. We would try to design a society where one can do the most basic thing there is and that is to live. The starting would have to be that those in the womb, who are coming into the world, would have a chance to be born. They would at least have a chance to make it into the world and would not be rudely interrupted in the womb by our own hand. This is simply the starting point upon which we could build a just society.

Rawls claims that because we already know our status in life, we are biased toward our position. I think this is true of many, especially when asked to think about abortion. Ronald Reagan wryly observed, "I've noticed that everyone who is for abortion has already been born." And this quip is in a way an appeal to the Rawlsian argument. It is a way of saying, "Gee, now that you've been born, it's very easy to selfishly declare that those who have not been born can be killed at will. It's easy to take away their freedom." We must remember that this isn't simply a thought experiment since every one of us was once a fetus. We all were in that position at one point. So as a former fetus, I oppose abortion. We all should. Barack Obama said, "If my daughters make a mistake, I don't want them punished with a baby." But what if your daughter was that baby? This argument only works when you know that you're in the position of the stronger, not the weaker, party.

We sometimes hear of people who have reached the top kicking the ladder out from under them. They've already gotten to the top. They don't care about the ladder anymore. Why? Because they've made it, and so goodbye ladder. Let everybody else fend for themselves at this point. Those who argue that being aborted is your bad luck somehow think that by caring about unborn babies you are caring less about a different group of people. But, of course, this is not the case because these things are not mutually exclusive. If we don't care about this injustice, abortion, one of the biggest injustices in the world in terms of numbers, a genocide beyond measure, why care about other injustices? Why try to solve hunger? Why fight racial discrimination? Why try to cure disease?

I condemn the "shrug your shoulders, throw up your hands" attitude. If we left everything to luck, we would never invent anything new, think anything new, or do anything of consequence. We would live in a society where the strongest people always overpower the weaker ones and civilization would be dramatically set back. To say it's fair for someone to be aborted, to be tortured, just assumes that you're not the one being tortured. And you're not. You will never be in the womb again, it's true, you're not the one being aborted. I realize that it's tempting to shrug your shoulders and feel like "it sucks for you" as long as it's not you.

This is no way for a decent civilized society to think. This is not the way that we should think. Life does suck in many ways, I am not denying it, but let's work hard to make it suck less, and one way to do that is to reduce the outrageous killing of the innocent, the killing that is abortion.

"Long is the way and hard, that out of Hell leads up to light."

—JOHN MILTON, *Paradise Lost*[348]

It's time to take stock of our situation. If it is true that there have been sixty-one million abortions in America alone since *Roe v. Wade*, then we have seen in this country, right in front of us, the greatest genocide in modern history. If we look at the last century, we see a succession of horrific mass killings. Pol Pot, the communist dictator of Cambodia, is responsible for the deaths of over 1.7 million people. The big three dictators of the twentieth century—Adolf Hitler, Joseph Stalin, and Mao Zedong of Communist China—killed far more. Hitler killed thirty million, including six million Jews. Stalin killed forty million, and Mao killed up to sixty million Chinese in his rampage of mass killing.[349] It is not only disheartening but terrifying to consider that this extreme level of mass killing has been occurring in America. What's even worse is that mass killings in other countries were perpetrated by a group of fanatical killers motivated by a destructive and insane ideology. In the case of the Holocaust, for example, the ideology of Nazism. It was Hitler, his SS men, and his troops who carried out this mass killing.

In this country, however, we have turned ordinary people into killers. One might almost say that we have privatized killing. It's not the state that comes in and executes people. It's that the state empowers women and couples to consult and make life-and-death decisions involving other people, other human beings. Now, as then, dehumanization is the key. The denial of the humanity of the victim is the prelude to executing the victim. We also have now, as then, some element of blaming the victim. The victim is in the way; the victim is a nuisance. The victim is a threat to society. The idea that the victim "needs to be terminated" is part of a vocabulary of dehumanization. Pro-choicers say, "We're not pro-abortion, we're pro-choice. We're not for killing, we're only for the option to kill. And we're not really killing at all, we are merely terminating a pregnancy."

This is Orwellian language intended to numb our senses and make us turn our eyes and, more importantly, our conscience away from what is going on in our country. Abortion corrupts. It corrupts the individual, it corrupts the family, and it corrupts the community, just as slavery did. And this makes it, in my view, the most urgent issue of our time. There are many other important issues. The economy is important. Terrorism is an important issue. Immigration and the border are important issues. But nothing is more important than ending the mass killing of human beings that is occurring today in a free society, in a democratic environment, and with the support of a party that calls itself democratic. This is evil. And this must stop. Now, will it stop?

I think the answer to that question is: It depends. In today's environment, the way for abortion to stop is through a single path. And that path leads straight to the United States Supreme Court. There's really no other way for abortion to stop, at least to stop it as a matter of law. It does no good today, ultimately, for a state to pass a law against abortion because the Supreme Court will strike it down. There is no point in having Congress pass a law against abortion and having the president sign it. It would be held unconstitutional as a trespass on *Roe v. Wade* and subsequent decisions along the same lines. So, everything depends on the court, and everything that follows depends on what happens to *Roe v. Wade*.

The Supreme Court currently seems to be precariously balanced five to four, with Chief Justice Roberts as a swing vote. I say he is a "swing vote" because while he is somewhat conservative, he has voted in favor of pro-choice decisions in the past, siding with the liberal judges on the Court. Unfortunately, Chief Justice Roberts is not across-the-board conservative, unlike the Democrat appointees, who are all across-the-board liberal. There seem to be four strong conservative votes that would incline against *Roe* and four strong liberal votes that would be in favor of *Roe v. Wade*. And so, if a vote were to be held today, it is impossible to predict an outcome. If the Left is able to appoint the next justice, or two, *Roe* will definitely remain intact for at least another generation. In the words of National Constitution Center president Jeffrey Rosen, "the pro-choice majority asks nominees to swear allegiance to the decision without being able to identify an intelligible principle to support it."[350]

Of course, if President Trump is able to appoint perhaps one, and possibly two, new justices, these nominations would cause a firestorm because the Left already knows what is at stake—that *Roe v. Wade* is in constitutional jeopardy. If *Roe v. Wade* is overturned now or in the reasonable future, there will be a cataclysm in this country. The Left will go berserk. We will have activists showing up at state legislatures and screaming, blocking entrances, perhaps throwing blood at legislators.

There will be a deafening scream, if you will, in favor of upholding abortion. And I think that this sight, people ultimately shrieking for the right to kill other people, is reminiscent of a kind of slave auction, where people shout out prices for the purchase of other human beings. But this is coming, and the pro-life movement needs to be ready for it. When I attend pro-life events and I see gentle people hoping, as they have for a generation now, for an overturning of *Roe*, I worry that not all are emotionally ready for the storm that is sure to come.

Pro-lifers mostly worry about losing in the courts, but are they ready to win in the courts? Toughening of pro-life nerve is needed. It's needed because the Left will make a supreme effort, if *Roe v. Wade* is overturned, to take the doctrine of *Roe*, which is abortion over the entire nine months, and try to ensure that every state in the country has a law that recognizes this right. It is logical to think the pro-abortion forces would work to transfer the present legal authority from the Supreme Court to the state legislature. This would mean taking something that was previously upheld solely by federal judicial fiat and now have it ratified through the democratic process in the country. If the pro-choice movement is successful in doing that, it will be a crushing defeat for the pro-life cause. In fact, it will make abortion more secure in the future than it has been in the past. It will give the support of democratic affirmation to something that had otherwise been upheld solely by, you might say, the votes of nine justices.

And so, this is an outcome that the pro-life movement must prevent. The pro-life movement must do more than champion the overturning of *Roe*, it must also support pro-life decision making at the congressional level, at the state level, and also in popular sentiment. The good news here is that more and more Americans are becoming pro-life. The political momentum today is clearly with the pro-life side—considering that various states are passing restrictions on abortion and the Left is fighting them at every turn. The pro-life movement is on the offense, and the pro-choice and pro-abortion movements are on the defense.

Technology is helping illuminate the horror of abortion. Young people are less willing to succumb to the Orwellian doublespeak of their parents. They are more realistic at looking at life, including unborn life, squarely in the eye, so to speak. They want to call a spade a spade. I think young people who support abortion are more likely to say, "Yes, it is killing human beings, but we think it's defensible under certain circumstances." But the idea that abortion is not killing, that mass killing is not going on, that fallacious illusion is no longer acceptable in America in the twenty-first century. I hope that these thoughts are a prelude to understanding what needs to happen.

The best chance for success, I think, is to envision the fight in progressive stages. The first stage perhaps is the limiting of the reach of *Roe*. So, this is a way of chipping away at *Roe* very much in the way that the civil rights movement in the 1930s but more in the 1940s and 1950s pushed to limit the reach of segregation. It didn't challenge segregation per se but found ways to knock out, one by one, the supports of segregation. Ultimately, the edifice of segregation itself collapsed. This reasoning would call for limiting *Roe* as the first step. And that's what the states are trying to do in passing laws like heartbeat bills, which call for restrictions on abortion after the child's heartbeat is detected. If those laws are upheld, they represent limitations on *Roe*.

The second step is overturning *Roe*, keeping in mind that overturning it does not end abortion. What it does is to relegate abortion law away from the courts and to the states. This means that each state would have a chance to vote up or down on abortion. Each state would decide if it wants to have regulations on abortion, allow abortion, or abolish abortion. And, in a sense, we would return to what, in the slavery context, Stephen Douglas called "popular sovereignty." What Douglas meant is that each community would decide for itself if slavery should be allowed or forbidden. That same logic would apply to abortion.

We can expect that some states would allow abortion to continue. New York and California, for example, would probably adopt laws very similar to *Roe*. Other states would place restrictions on abortion, and some states would eliminate abortion altogether. This process would be a great improvement over what we have now. The overturning of *Roe* has been the hope of the pro-life movement since 1973. We should continue to push for this, and it will be a great victory when it occurs.

But the third step would be a federal ban on abortion that would make abortion illegal throughout the country. There might be narrow exceptions: exceptions perhaps for rape, incest, or to save the life of the mother. But aside from those rare cases, abortion would cease to be lawful in America.

Notice that these three steps closely mirror what actually happened with slavery. Initially, the Republican Party in the 1860 election tried to prevent the extension of slavery. The second step was for slavery to become illegal in certain states but legal in others. Basically, all the northern states adopted laws that moved toward getting rid of slavery. Southern states, on the other hand, upheld slavery. The third step was a federal ban on slavery enshrined by amendments in the Constitution itself.

I would like to see a constitutional amendment upholding the right to life. I recognize that such an amendment would be very difficult to pass not only in the current political environment but even in the foreseeable future. Short of a constitutional amendment, however, abortion can be eliminated legally through a federal ban, which is not unthinkable. That would require a Republican majority in the House and in the Senate and a Republican president, supported by a Supreme Court that is pro-life. Those things are not inconceivable, not just in the distant future but in the near future. And this is why, for those of us who are pro-life, this is a moment of anticipation and electrifying excitement. *Roe v. Wade* can be overturned. That's the critical step. And that's happened before with segregation. Let's remember that the Supreme Court in 1954 in the *Brown v. Board of Education* decision knocked out a segregation law, a segregation decision, *Plessy v. Ferguson*, which had existed for over fifty years going back to the end of the nineteenth century.

For a long time, courts had upheld *Plessy v. Ferguson*, but in the *Brown* decision, the court simply looked at the separate but equal doctrine and basically said separate is not equal. And we are looking now for a similar decision, a lethal blow to *Roe v. Wade*, so it can join *Plessy* in the dustbin of history and in retrospect be seen as a relic of barbarism.

I've been talking about changes in the law, but I now want to talk about how law is upheld. Law is ultimately upheld by public sentiment and by culture. Plato famously said that the law is a teacher. And what he meant is that the law does two things simultaneously. It prevents things, but it also educates. It teaches people about what's right and what's wrong. For example, the fact that we have had civil rights laws on the books for almost half a century now has shown a younger generation of people that racism is not acceptable.

The law helps educate people in that. Of course, the law is not the only teacher, but it's difficult to have laws where people's sentiments are completely contrary to a law. For several years, for example, America had prohibition laws that forbade the sale and use of intoxicating drinks. But those laws were terribly unpopular. And when you have laws like that, the law in a sense becomes a joke because it's not supported by the people. We don't want abortion laws to go down this path. With abortion, we need to bring about a genuine change in sentiment across the nation. We need a cultural transformation that sees abortion in the same evil light that we see slavery today: as an evil. And so we have to ask ourselves, how do societies change in this way? Is such change even possible?

Yes, it is possible. Culture does change. I think for example, about America in the twentieth century. The novelist F. Scott Fitzgerald writes about the Jazz Age, the Roaring Twenties, which had a great deal of promiscuity. And all of this changed dramatically with a turn to moral restraint during the 1930s that continued into the 1940s and 1950s, the era of what we now call the greatest generation. Admittedly, this cultural change was a product of two important facts: the Depression and World War II.

Nevertheless, cultures change, and we have to ask how we can have such change today. What we are trying to do is to bring about a moral awakening, a moral awakening that touches the hearts of the great majority. I'm not sure that we're trying to persuade the bad guys. I'm not trying to persuade Planned Parenthood that it's in the wrong business. It's very difficult to persuade people like that. They're making a great deal of money on abortion.

This is like trying to persuade the slave owner that he should emancipate his slaves. Now, some slave owners did do that, particularly around the time of America's founding. Their conscience prevailed, you might say, over their pocketbook. And that can happen in some cases, but by and large, our target is to persuade the people in the middle. The people in the middle are uncertain and unconvinced, and to some degree they blow with the wind. They go with whichever side they think is cool. Such people are morally unreliable, but they are winnable.

We need to make it uncool to support abortion. We need to create a pro-life culture because the pro-life culture saves lives. We need to convince people who believe that abortion is the lesser evil that, in fact, it is the greater evil. We have a starting point with the people who say that abortion is a lesser evil in that they admit that abortion is an evil, otherwise they wouldn't call it a lesser evil; so it is an evil. And we have to build on that to help them understand that the evil represented by abortion is far greater than any so-called good that is obtained by ending this human life.

The abolitionists brought about a change of heart with regard to slavery, and they did so by appealing to both the head and the heart. They made rational arguments, legal and constitutional arguments, but they also told stories. I think, for example, of *Uncle Tom's Cabin*, a very influential book by Harriet Beecher Stowe. She once commented that she was not trying to make an argument; she was trying to paint a picture. She said, "You can argue with arguments. You can fight back ultimately, in a dispute, but you can't argue with a picture. You can't dispute a story. A story is going to ultimately sway your conscience and your emotion." And this, she says, is how we get the American people to awaken to the true horror of slavery.

And I think the same is true with abortion. Culture is malleable. What we want people to do is to recognize that an abortion culture is a destructive culture. It is a culture of harming people. Look at the way that there's been a change of heart in America over smoking cigarettes. Smoking cigarettes was once completely normal. It was preposterous to ask people to stop smoking or to smoke only in certain limited areas. It seemed inconceivable to get large numbers of people to put away their cigarettes because they didn't want to do it anymore. And yet this is exactly what has happened. We can't equate these two causes. Smoking is incomparably more trivial in importance than abortion, but nevertheless, it is an illuminating indicator of how cultures do change.

Turning away from abortion is also turning away from the abortionist. And the abortionist is a wicked figure in our culture today. The abortionist is the slave catcher of our time. Lincoln liked to comment to how the slave catcher was seen throughout society, even in the South, as a loathsome individual—as a kind of low character. Abortionists occupy exactly the same position. They are the sanctioned killers of our society. We need ultimately to highlight this. And there's nothing wrong with doing that. Just as the Left calls out racism and asks society and other people to denounce racists, we must ask society and others to denounce the killing of innocent babies.

We must be hard on the abortion industry and hard on the pro-choice and pro-abortion politicians who are ultimately the political backbone of the abortion industry. These are people who are propagating killing. They're blinding women and influencing them to do things that they would not otherwise do. And we must also demonize those who celebrate abortion. People who say abortion is a positive good are the modern-day equivalent of the people who said slavery is a positive good. There's a good deal of rationalization here as well as a good deal of sheer wickedness.

Anyone who thinks that ending another life is something to be celebrated is ultimately a morally bankrupt person, an evil person.

In the end, the evil is sustained not only by the wicked people but also by the people in the middle who succumb to base rationalizations. And perhaps the evilest of these rationalizations is the idea of "Who is to say what life is?" Yes, I might think that this is a life and killing is wrong, but you might feel differently; therefore, I should step back and not act on my belief. When we're dealing with life, we know what life is. We know what human life is. We know what is happening inside the womb. We can see it. And we should not turn away from what we can see or pretend that other people are seeing something different.

They are seeing exactly what we see. They know exactly what we know. And there is no need to succumb to the base relativism of pretending because it is a bad pretense—that life, the existence of other emerging developing human beings, is somehow solely in the eye of the beholder. It's not. These are human lives. Purposefully killing them is wrong. And we need to awaken our society to it.

Sometimes I think that we need a spiritual awakening for the full recognition of this to take place. America has had those before. Moments of great religious and spiritual revival have in fact preceded pivotal events of our history. The first great awakening came right before the Revolutionary War. The second great awakening came before and then continued after the Civil War. These represent people turning to God, not merely to anticipate the next life but also to do a sort of reevaluation, a reassessment of how things are in the world now. This realization helps people reconsider matters that they previously thought were settled and to produce not only a conversion of society but also an inner, personal conversion.

The line between good and evil doesn't run just between us and them. It runs through every human heart. We should work to produce a change of heart of this sort that will mobilize the religious community toward the pro-life cause in a much more active way. Also we should mobilize people toward a call to God, or in some cases to conscience, so that what is right triumphs over what is merely convenient.

What I've described in this book shouldn't just make us aghast. It should make us want to do more. It should make us use our influence to demand legal change and to work for a cultural change. This can be done by speaking out, by using social media, by joining grassroots movements to fight against abortion, and also by joining movements to help women in need. Helping struggling women is very meaningful. Every woman having a baby needs a support system—someone to also share their joys and sorrows. There's so much that we can do for others. And we can also support charities that help children in need. Ultimately, the pro-life cause is the cause of conscience. It is the cause of the caring heart.

America is a society that has lost its moorings on this issue. We have allowed mass killing to become normalized. This is not the society our Founders sought to create. We have become in a sense unworthy of our noble origins. We affirm the rights that have been given to us by our Creator, but we desecrate those rights and we dishonor our Creator by permitting this scandal to exist in our midst. Working together, however, we can open eyes and hearts to what is going on. We can mobilize political support for change. We can work for cultural renewal and moral renewal and spiritual renewal. And together we can end the scourge of abortion in America.

I would like to end this book, *The Choice*, by saying that you have the choice. In America, you can make a choice about whether to have an abortion today, but you can also make a choice about whether you will join this cause, the pro-life movement. Life is full of choices. So, I ask you—What is your choice? Do you make the choice to take a stand for the voiceless? As Jesus asks, "Who do you say I am?" we can almost think of the fetus asking us, "Who do you say I am?" Do you answer cluster of cells or person with dignity? But I also ask you, the reader, "Who do you say you are?" We cannot say we are good or merciful if we live our lives as coldhearted people devoid of any love for others. It is often our choices that define us. Mother Teresa said, "Do things for people not because of who they are or what they do in return, but because of who you are." You can define who you are by making a choice here. You may never be repaid for it. But anytime we are called to take a stand, hanging out with friends, or casting our vote, we make a choice, and it reflects our character. What will yours be?

NOTES

1. Stephen Dinan, "Kavanaugh Accuser Admits to Making Up Rape Accusation as 'Tactic,' " Global News, November 3, 2018, https://globalnews.ca/news/462 8088/brett-kavanaugh-rape-accusation-lie/.

2. Mollie Hemingway, "Blasey Ford Attorney Admits Abortion Support 'Motivated' Anti-Kavanaugh Accusations," *The Federalist*, September 4, 2019, https:// thefederalist.com /2019/09/04/blasey-ford-attorney-admits-abortion-supported-motivated-anti-kavanaugh-accusations/.

3. Benjamin Fearnow, "Video Shows Christine Blasey Ford's Attorney Saying Kavanaugh Testimony Was Politically Motivated," *Newsweek*, September 8, 2019, https://www.newsweek .com/christine-blasey-ford-attorney-debra-katz-roe-v-wade-video-politically-motivated-testimony-1458217.

4. Harry Jaffa, *A New Birth of Freedom: Abraham Lincoln and The Coming of the Civil War* (Lanham: Rowman and Littlefield Publishers Inc., 2004), 247–248.

5. WSJ Editorial Board, "Schumer Threatens the Court," *Wall Street Journal*, March 4, 2020 https://www.wsj.com/articles/schumer-threatens-the-court-11583368462.

6. Editorial Board, "Schumer Threatens the Court."

7. Adam Liptak, "John Roberts Condemns Schumer for Saying Justices 'Will Pay the Price' for 'Awful Decisions,' " *New York Times*, March 4, 2020, https://www.nytimes .com/2020/03/04/us/roberts-schumer-supreme-court.html.

8. NY Governor's Office, "Governor Cuomo Directs One World Trade Center and Other Landmarks to be Lit in Pink to Celebrate Signing of the Reproductive Health Act," January 22, 2019, https://www.governor.ny.gov/news/governor-cuomo-directs-one-world-trade-center-and-other-landmarks-be-lit-pink-celebrate-signing.

9. Ibid.

10. Chanshimla Varah, "Abortion The Silent Killer of 2018, Total Death Amounts to Over 41 Million," *News Nation*, January 4, 2019, https://english.newsnationtv.com/lifestyle /health-and-fitness/abortion-legalised-abortion-unplanned-baby-the-silent-killer-of-2018-total-death-amounts-to-nearly-41-million-210543.html.

11. Amelia Bonow, "How One Woman Became an Activist With the Hashtag #ShoutYour-Abortion," Oprah.com, http://www.oprah.com/inspiration/how-one-woman-became-an-activist-with-the-hashtag-shoutyourabortion_1#ixzz6TYD1SBk5.

12. Thomas Jefferson, Letter to John Holmes, https://www.loc.gov/exhibits/jefferson /159.html.

13. William Shakespeare, "Hamlet," Act 3, Scene 1 (Norwalk, Connecticut: Easton Press, 1992), 59.

NOTES

14. Richard Stith, "Nominal Babies," *First Things*, February, 1999, https://www.firstthings.com/article/1999/02/001-nominal-babies.

15. *Merriam-Webster.com Dictionary*, s.v. "Pregnant," accessed June 16, 2020, https://www.merriam-webster.com/dictionary/pregnant.

16. Guttmacher Institute, FAQ Page, https://www.guttmacher.org/guttmacher-institute-faq.

17. Rachel Benson Gold, "The Implications of Defining When a Woman Is Pregnant," Guttmacher Institute, May 9, 2005, https://www.guttmacher.org/gpr/2005/05/implications-defining-when-woman-pregnant.

18. Ashley Strickland, "Water Detected in Atmosphere of Potentially Habitable Super-Earth," *CNN*, September 11, 2019, https://www.cnn.com/2019/09/11/world/water-atmosphere-exoplanet-scn/index.html.

19. Seti Institute, Mission, https://www.seti.org/about-us/mission.

20. "Lesson 1: The 7 Characteristics of Life," Portland Community College, http://spot.pcc.edu/~jvolpe/b/bi112/lec/examples/112examplesCh1_Ch3.htm.

21. Randy Alcorn, "Fully Human From The Beginning," Eternal Perspective Ministries, November 30, 2011, https://www.epm.org/blog/2011/Nov/30/fully-human-beginning.

22. Mitch Leslie, "Biologists Create The Most Lifelike Artificial Cells Yet," *Science*, November 18, 2019, https://www.sciencemag.org/news/2018/11/biologists-create-most-lifelike-artificial-cells-yet.

23. Ibid.

24. Christopher Chow, Encyclopedia Britannica, "Cell," accessed July 14, 2020, https://www.britannica.com/science/cell-biology.

25. "What is a Cell?" U.S. National Library of Medicine, July 28 2020, https://ghr.nlm.nih.gov/primer/basics/cell#:~:text=Cells%20are%20the%20basic%20building,and%20carry%20out%20specialized%20functions.

26. Fred de Miranda, MD (updated by Patricia Lee June, MD), American College of Pediatricians, "When Human Life Begins," March 2017.

27. American College of Pediatricians, "When Human Life Begins."

28. Anne Casselman, "Identical Twins' Genes Are Not Identical," Scientific American, April 3, 2008, https://www.scientificamerican.com/article/identical-twins-genes-are-not-identical/.

29. American College of Pediatricians, "When Human Life Begins."

30. Ibid.

31. "Life Begins at Fertilization," Princeton.edu, https://www.princeton.edu/~prolife/articles/embryoquotes2.html.

32. Mayo Clinic Staff, "Fetal Development: The 1st Trimester," Mayo Clinic, June 30, 2020, https://www.mayoclinic.org/healthy-lifestyle/pregnancy-week-by-week/in-depth/prenatal-care/art-20045302.

33. Life Matters Worldwide, "When Does Life Begin?," https://www.lifemattersww.org/Need-Help/Questions-about-abortion/When-Does-Life-Begin.

34. R. C. Sproul, *Abortion: A Rational Look at an Emotional Issue* (Orlando, FL: Reformation Trust: A Division of Ligonier Ministries, 2010), 54.

35. Life Matters Worldwide, "When Does Life Begin?"

36. Sproul, *Abortion: A Rational Look at an Emotional Issue*, 54.

37. Life Matters Worldwide, "When Does Life Begin?"

38. Ibid.

39. Ibid.

40. Sproul, *Abortion: A Rational Look at an Emotional Issue*, 54.

NOTES

41. William Wordsworth, "The French Revolution As It Appeared to Enthusiasts At Its Commencement," 1809, https://www.poetryfoundation.org/poems/45518/the-french-revolution-as-it-appeared-to-enthusiasts-at-its-commencement.

42. Shane Trejo, "British Academics Produce Research Indicating That Fetuses May Feel Pain After 13 Weeks," *Big League Politics*, January 21, 2020, https://bigleaguepolitics.com/british-academics-produce-research-indicating-that-fetuses-may-feel-pain-after-13-weeks/.

43. "Beware High Levels of Cortisol, the Stress Hormone," *Premier Health*, February 5, 2017, https://www.premierhealth.com/your-health/articles/women-wisdom-wellness-/beware-high-levels-of-cortisol-the-stress-hormone.

44. Pam Belluck, "Complex Science at Issue in Politics of Fetal Pain," *New York Times*, September 6, 2013, https://www.nytimes.com/2013/09/17/health/complex-science-at-issue-in-politics-of-fetal-pain.html.

45. Ibid.

46. Ibid.

47. Dr. Bjorn Merker, quoted in Belluck, "Complex Science at Issue in Politics of Fetal Pain.

48. Stuart Derbyshire and John C. Bockmann, "Reconsidering Fetal Pain," *Journal of Medical Ethics*, 46 (2020): 3–6, https://jme.bmj.com/content/46/1/3.

49. Ibid., 3.

50. Shane Trejo, "British Academics Produce Research Indicating That Fetuses May Feel Pain After 13 Weeks."

51. Heidi Murkoff, *What to Expect When You're Expecting*, 5th ed. (New York: Workman, 2016), 212.

52. Ibid.

53. Kanwaljeet Anand, quoted in Belluck, "Complex Science at Issue in Politics of Fetal Pain."

54. Shane Trejo, "British Academics Produce Research Indicating That Fetuses May Feel Pain After 13 Weeks."

55. Michael S. Gazzaniga, "The Ethical Brain," *New York Times*, June 19, 2005, https://www.nytimes.com/2005/06/19/books/chapters/the-ethical-brain.html.

56. "When Does the Fetus's Brain Begin to Work?" Zero to Three, https://www.zerotothree.org/resources/1375-when-does-the-fetus-s-brain-begin-to-work.

57. Murkoff, *What to Expect When You're Expecting*, 157.

58. Ibid.

59. The Fertility Center, "Baby Prep: The Importance of Talking to Your Baby in the Womb," September 21, 2016, https://fertilitycenterlv.com/blog/pregnancy/baby-prep-the-importance-of-talking-to-your-baby-in-the-womb/.

60. James Barrett, "'The View' Gasps at Ben Carson's Defense of Unborn Babies," *Daily Wire*, October 7, 2015, https://www.dailywire.com/news/view-gasps-ben-carsons-defense-unborn-babies-james-barrett.

61. Nancy Shute, "Beyond Birth: A Child's Cells May Help or Harm the Mother Long after Delivery," *Scientific American*, April 30, 2010, https://www.scientificamerican.com/article/fetal-cells-microchimerism/.

62. Ibid.

63. Ibid.

64. Stephanie Pritchard and Diana W. Bianchi, "Fetal Cell Microchimerism in the Maternal Heart: Baby Gives Back," *Circulation Research* 110, no. 1 (2012): 3–5, AHA Journals, January 6, 2012, https://doi.org/10.1161/CIRCRESAHA.111.260299.

65. "Ethics Guide: When Is the Foetus 'Alive'?" BBC.com, 2014, http://www.bbc.co.uk/ethics/abortion/child/alive_1.shtml.

66. "Some Thoughts on Autonomy and Equality in Relation to *Roe v. Wade*," excerpted from 63 N.C.L. REV 375 (1985).

67. Democratic Party Platform, "Ensure the Health and Safety of all Americans: Securing Reproductive Health, Rights, and Justice," 2020, https://democrats.org/where-we-stand/party-platform/ensure-the-health-and-safety-of-all-americans/.

68. Sproul, "Abortion: A Rational Look at an Emotional Issue," 55.

69. Ibid., 56.

70. BBC, "Ethics Guide: When Is the Foetus 'Alive'?"

71. Peter Singer, *Rethinking Life and Death: The Collapse of Our Traditional Ethics* (New York: St. Martin's Griffin, 1994), 217.

72. EWTN, "Ben Shapiro Responds to Abortion Claims," *YouTube*, October 19, 2017, https://www.youtube.com/watch?v=ezZDegitDgo.

73. Alan Rappeport, "Hillary Clinton Roundly Criticized for Referring to the Unborn as a 'Person,'" *New York Times*, April 4, 2016, https://www.nytimes.com/politics/first-draft/2016/04/04/hillary-clinton-roundly-criticized-for-referring-to-the-unborn-as-a-person/.

74. The Hippocratic Oath, U.S. National Library of Medicine, https://www.nlm.nih.gov/hmd/greek/greek_oath.html.

75. Bernie Sanders (@BernieSanders), Twitter, January 24, 2020, 9:28 a.m., https://twitter.com/berniesanders/status/1220760231061413890?lang=en.

76. Josh Shapiro (@PAAttorneyGen), Twitter, January 9, 2020, 6:12 a.m., https://twitter.com/paattorneygen/status/1215275032093646850?s=11.

77. "What Facts About Abortion Do I Need to Know," *Planned Parenthood*, https://www.plannedparenthood.org/learn/abortion/considering-abortion/what-facts-about-abortion-do-i-need-know.

78. "Safety of Abortion," *National Abortion Federation*, https://prochoice.org/wp-content/uploads/safety_of_abortion.pdf.

79. CAP Women (@CAPwomen), Twitter, February 4, 2020, https://twitter.com/capwomen/status/1224890032860864513?s=11.

80. Steven Ertelt, "Abortion Backers Oppose Regulations That Could Have Stopped Gosnell," *Life News*, April 18, 2013, https://www.lifenews.com/2013/04/18/abortion-backers-oppose-regulations-that-could-have-stopped-gosnell/.

81. Ibid.

82. Ibid.

83. Miriam Berg, "These 4 Types of TRAP Laws are Dangerously Chipping Away at Abortion Access Under the Guise of 'Women's Health,'" *Planned Parenthood*, June 15, 2016, https://www.plannedparenthoodaction.org/blog/these-4-types-of-trap-laws-are-dangerously-chipping-away-abortion-access-under-the-guise-of-womens-health.

84. June Medical Services L. L. C. Et Al. V. Russo, Interim Secretary, Louisiana Department of Health and Hospitals, Supreme Court of the United States, Decided June 29, 2020, https://www.supremecourt.gov/opinions/19pdf/18-1323_c07d.pdf.

85. "In-Clinic Abortion Procedures," *Planned Parenthood*, https://www.plannedparenthood.org/learn/abortion/in-clinic-abortion-procedures.

86. "Reproductive Health Data and Statistics," *Center for Disease Control and Prevention*, https://www.cdc.gov/reproductivehealth/data_stats/.

87. "How Does the Abortion Pill Work," *Planned Parenthood*, https://www.plannedparenthood.org/learn/abortion/the-abortion-pill/how-does-the-abortion-pill-work.

88. Gina Kolata, "France and China Allow Sale of a Drug For Early Abortion," *New York Times*, September 24, 1988, https://www.nytimes.com/1988/09/24/us/france-and-china-allow -sale-of-a-drug-for-early-abortion.html.

89. CRS Report for Congress, "Abortion: Termination of an Early Pregnancy with RU-486 (Mifepristone)," February 23, 2001, https://www.everycrsreport.com/reports/RL30866 .html.

90. MIFEPREX (mifepristone) tablets Label, https://www.accessdata.fda.gov /drugsatfda_docs/label/2016/020687s020lbl.pdf.

91. "The Abortion Pill," *Planned Parenthood*, https://www.plannedparenthood.org /learn/abortion/the-abortion-pill.

92. "Abortion Procedures," Abort 73.com, https://abort73.com/abortion/abortion _techniques/.

93. Sarah Terzo, "Pro-choice woman recounts 'emotionally scary and dangerous' experience with abortion pill," *Live Action*, May 9, 2017, https://www.liveaction.org/news /pro-choice-woman-recounts-emotionally-scary-dangerous-experience-with-abortion-pill/.

94. Hayley Macmillen, "Here's What It's Really Like to Take the Abortion Pill," *Cosmopolitan*, October 3, 2016, https://www.cosmopolitan.com/sex-love/a3389296/abortion-pill -mifeprex-mifepristone/.

95. Ibid.

96. MIFEPREX (mifepristone) tablets Label, https://www.accessdata.fda.gov/drugsatfda _docs/label/2016/020687s020lbl.pdf.

97. Ibid.

98. Dr. Jen Gunter, "What is the 'Mexican abortion pill' and how safe is it?" July 27, 2013, https://drjengunter.com/2013/07/27/what-is-the-mexican-abortion-pill-and-how-safe-is-it/.

99. "Abortion Procedures," Abort73, https://abort73.com/abortion/abortion_techniques/.

100. Ibid.

101. Ibid.

102. Ibid.

103. Murkoff, *What to Expect When You're Expecting*, 261.

104. Ibid., 247.

105. Living Waters, "Ex-Abortion Doctor Tells The Shocking Truth About Abortion," *YouTube*, February 5, 2019, https://www.youtube.com/watch?v=A16gzm9eaa8.

106. Ibid.

107. Linda A. Bartlett et al., "Risk Factors for Legal Induced Abortion–Related Mortality in the United States," *Obstetrics & Gynecology* 103, no. 4 (2004): 729–737, http://www.ncbi .nlm.nih.gov/pubmed/15051566.

108. "Abortion Procedures," *Live Action*, https://www.abortionprocedures.com/?__hstc =61024563.441a468c0%20e350739f67022ecfb826c24.1578349109614.1578939531064 .1578942861415%20.3&__hssc=61024563.1.1578942861415&__hsfp=1269184093 #1466802055946%20-992e6a14-9b1d.

109. Patricia A. Lohr, "Surgical Abortion in Second Trimester," *Reproductive Health Matters* 16, suppl. 31 (2008): 156, www.ncbi.nlm.nih.gov/pubmed/18772096.

110. Cassy Fiano-Chesser, "Do Saline Abortions, Where Babies Are Burned in Salt, Still Happen in the U.S.?" *Live Action*, November 30, 2016, https://www.liveaction.org/news /saline-abortions-still-happen-america/.

111. P. D. Darney et al., "Digoxin to Facilitate Late Second-Trimester Abortion: A Randomized, Masked, Placebo-Controlled Trial," *Obstetrics and Gynecology* 97, no. 3 (2001): 471–476, www.ncbi.nlm.nih.gov/pubmed/11239659.

NOTES

112. Richard Selzer, "What I Saw at the Abortion," *Esquire*, January 1, 1976, https://archive.esquire.com/article/1976/1/1/what-i-saw-at-the-abortion.

113. David M. Fergusson, with Joseph M. Boden and L. John Harwood, "Does Abortion Reduce the Mental Health Risks of Unwanted or Unintended Pregnancy? A Re-appraisal of the Evidence," *Australian & New Zealand Journal of Psychiatry* 47, no. 9 (2013): 819–827.

114. Ryan Jaslow, "Abortion Tied to Sharp Decline in Women's Mental Health," *CBS News*, September 1, 2011, https://www.cbsnews.com/news/abortion-tied-to-sharp-decline-in-womens-mental-health/.

115. Ibid.

116. SBC staff, "Healing the Wounds of Abortion," *SBC Life*, January 1, 2003, http://www.sbclife.net/article/946/healing-the-wounds-of-abortion.

117. John Hart Ely, "The Wages of Crying Wolf: A Comment on Roe v. Wade," 947, Yale Law School Legal Scholarship Repository.

118. Roe v. Wade, 410 U.S. 113 (1973), https://supreme.justia.com/cases/federal/us/410/113/.

119. Paul Gewirtz, "The Jurisprudence of Hypotheticals," excerpted from 32 J. Legal Educ. 120 (1982).

120. Laurence H. Tribe, "The Supreme Court, 1972 Term—Foreword: Toward a Model of Roles in the Due Process of Life and Law," *Harvard Law Review* 87, no. 1 (1973): 7.

121. Daniel K. Williams, "The Real Reason to Criticize Roe," *Public Discourse*, January 24, 2013, https://www.thepublicdiscourse.com/2013/01/7679/.

122. Robert Bork, "The Tempting of America" (New York: Free Press, 1990), 111–116, 264–265.

123. Ruth B. Ginsburg, "Some Thoughts on Autonomy and Equality in Relation to Roe v. Wade," 63 N.C.L. REV. 375 (1985), http://scholarship.law.unc.edu/nclr/vol63/iss2/4.

124. Roe v. Wade, 410 U.S. 113 (1973).

125. Michael McConnell, *How Not To Promote Serious Deliberation About Abortion*, excerpted from *University of Chicago Law Review* 58 (1991): 1181, 1187–1188, 1189–1190, 1198.

126. Clarke D. Forsythe, "Abuse of Discretion: Inside the Story of Roe v. Wade" (New York: Encounter Books, 2013), 9.

127. Justice White, "Dissent, Roe v. Wade, US Supreme Court," C-Span, http://landmarkcases.c-span.org/pdf/Roe_White_Dissent.pdf.

128. Ibid.

129. Business Insider, "ALAN DERSHOWITZ: Why Supreme Court got Roe v. Wade wrong," *YouTube*, November 4, 2016, https://www.youtube.com/watch?v=_yAcf-S1wEU.

130. Alexis de Tocqueville, *Democracy in America* (New York: Vintage Books, 1990) Volume I, 244.

131. Emma Green, "Why Democrats Ditched the Hyde Amendment," *The Atlantic*, June 14, 2019, https://www.theatlantic.com/politics/archive/2019/06/democrats-hyde-amendment-history/591646/.

132. Bernie Sanders (@BernieSanders), Twitter, Jun 5, 2019, 7:54 a.m., https://twitter.com/berniesanders/status/1136285225632370688?la.

133. Tara Law, "Joe Biden Dropped His Support for the Hyde Amendment. Here's How It Became a Flashpoint on Abortion," Time, June 7, 2019, https://time.com/5603055/hyde-amendment-abortion-joe-biden/.

134. Kirsten Gillibrand (@SenGillibrand), Twitter, June 5, 2019, 9:34 a.m., https://twitter.com/sengillibrand/status/1136310247944052743?la.

135. Cory Booker (@CoryBooker), Twitter, June 5, 2019, 1:30 p.m., https://twitter .com/corybooker/status/1136369803822817280?lang=en.

136. Charlie Spiering, Pete Buttigieg: " 'We Are All Lifted Up' by Stories About Abortions," *Breitbart*, February 17, 2020, https://www.breitbart.com/politics/2020/02/17/pete-buttigieg -we-are-all-lifted-up-by-stories-about-abortions/.

137. Katie Glueck, "Joe Biden Denounces Hyde Amendment, Reversing His Position," *New York Times*, June 6, 2019, https://www.nytimes.com/2019/06/06/us/politics/joe-biden-hyde -amendment.html.

138. Rachel del Guidice, "6 Things to Know About the Hyde Amendment," *The Daily Signal*, June 7, 2019, https://www.dailysignal.com/2019/06/07/6-things-to-know-about-the -hyde-amendment/.

139. Ibid.

140. John Stuart Mill, *On Liberty* (Indianapolis: Hackett Publishing, 1978), 12.

141. Slate staff, "The Abortions We Don't Talk About," *Slate*, July 29, 2018, https:// slate.com/human-interest/2018/07/the-abortions-we-dont-talk-about-six-slate-women-tell -their-stories.htm.

142. Ibid.

143. Mill, *On Liberty*, 53.

144. Rand Paul, "Advocating for the Sanctity of Life," https://www.paul.senate.gov/issues /advocating-sanctity-life.

145. Harry Jaffa, *Crisis of the House Divided: An Interpretation of the Issues in the Lincoln-Douglas Debates* (Chicago: University of Chicago Press, 2009).

146. Abraham Lincoln April 18, 1864 in "Address at Sanity Fair," Baltimore, Maryland, in "Selected Speeches and Writings By Abraham Lincoln" (New York: Vintage Books, 1992), 422–423.

147. Jake Johnson, "Come 'Say This to My Face,' Says Ayanna Pressley After Betsy DeVos Compares Being Pro-Choice to Being Pro-Slavery," *Common Dreams*, January 24, 2020, https:// www.commondreams.org/news/2020/01/24/come-say-my-face-says-ayanna-pressley-after -betsy-devos-compares-being-pro-choice.

148. Naomi Wolf, "Naomi Wolf on Abortion: 'Our Bodies, Our Souls,' " *New Statesman*, January 27, 2013, https://www.newstatesman.com/politics/politics/2013/01/naomi-wolf -abortion-our-bodies-our-souls.

149. Brad Allen, "The Government Approved a Death Certificate Confirming My Son Liam Was Killed in an Abortion," *Life News*, January 16, 2020, https://www.lifenews .com/2020/01/16/the-government-approved-a-death-certificate-confirming-my-son-liam -was-killed-in-an-abortion/.

150. Ashe Schow, "Ex-Husband Wins In Court, Prevents Wife From Using Frozen Embryos," *The Daily Wire*, January 31, 2020, https://www.dailywire.com/news/ex-husband-wins-in-court -prevents-wife-from-using-frozen-embryos.

151. Alexandra Bowman, "The Men Who Feel Left out of US Abortion Debate," *BBC*, August 28, 2019, https://www.bbc.com/news/world-us-canada-49240582.

152. Ibid.

153. William Shakespeare, "Hamlet," Act 2, Scene 2 (Norwalk, Connecticut: Easton Press, 1992), 47.

154. Katha Pollitt, "Reclaiming Abortion Rights," *Dissent Magazine*, Fall 2015, https:// www.dissentmagazine.org/article/reclaiming-abortion-rights-katha-pollitt.

155. Erika Bachiochi, "The Troubling Ideals at the Heart of Abortion Rights," *The Atlantic*, January 24, 2020, https://www.theatlantic.com/ideas/archive/2020/01/equality -autonomy-abortion/605356/.

NOTES

156. Stacey Tisdale, "Gloria Steinem on Patriarchy, Abortion and Economic Independence," *Al Jazeera*, July 12, 2019, https://www.aljazeera.com/ajimpact/gloria-steinem-talks-patriarchy-abortion-economic-independence-190712165559932.html.

157. Matt Donnelly, "Gloria Steinem Calls Trump's Anti-Abortion Rally Visit, Heartbeat Bills 'The Definition of Patriarchy,'" *Variety*, January 29, 2020, https://variety.com/2020/film/news/gloria-steinem-calls-trumps-anti-abortion-rally-visit-heartbeat-bills-the-definition-of-patriarchy-1203484348/.

158. Gloria Steinem, "If Men Could Menstruate," 1986, https://www.haverford.edu/psychology/ddavis/p109g/steinem.menstruate.html.

159. Ellen Willis, "Ellen Willis on Abortion," *The Village Voice*, March 8, 2019, Ellen Willis on Abortion, https://www.villagevoice.com/2019/03/08/ellen-willis-on-abortion/.

160. Gabriel Fernandes, "Feminismo Radical (1969), Shulamith Firestone," *YouTube*, October 15, 2018, https://www.youtube.com/watch?v=Owe3-bH61Oc.

161. William Shakespeare, "Measure for Measure," Act 2, Scene 2 (Norwalk, Connecticut: Easton Press, 1992), 29.

162. Sarah Burns, "'It saved my life': Thousands of Women Share Their Termination Stories to End Shame and Stigma as #ShoutYourAbortion hashtag Sweeps Twitter," *Daily Mail*, September 22, 2015, https://www.dailymail.co.uk/femail/article-3244385/Shout-Abortion-hashtag-trends-women-share-experiences-end-shame-stigma.html.

163. Shout Your Abortion, https://shoutyourabortion.com/.

164. Thank God for Abortion, https://www.thankgodforabortion.com/.

165. Obianuju Ekeocha (@obianuju), Twitter, November 14, 2019, https://twitter.com/obianuju/status/1195090669024546816?s=11.

166. Diane J. Cho, "27 Celebrities Who Have Shared Their Abortion Stories to Help Women Feel Less Alone," People.com, March 26, 2020, https://people.com/health/celebrity-abortion-stories-busy-philipps-jameela-jamil/.

167. Anne Cohen, "Michelle Williams Celebrates A Woman's Right To Choose In Passionate Golden Globes Speech," *Refinery* 29, January 25, 2020, https://www.refinery29.com/en-us/2020/01/9143968/michelle-williams-abortion-womens-rights-speech-golden-globes-2020.

168. Abby Gardner, "Michelle Williams Delivers Powerful Golden Globes Speech About a Woman's Right to Choose," *Glamour*, January 6, 2020, https://www.glamour.com/story/michelle-williams-speech-2020-golden-globes.

169. David Ng, "Hollywood Heaps Praise on Michelle Williams for Pro-Abortion Golden Globes Acceptance Speech," *Breitbart*, January 6, 2020, https://www.breitbart.com/entertainment/2020/01/06/hollywood-heaps-praise-on-michelle-williams-for-pro-abortion-golden-globes-acceptance-speech/.

170. Elizabeth Banks (@ElizabethBanks), Twitter, January 5, 2020, 7:15 p.m., https://twitter.com/elizabethbanks/status/1214022564973989888?lang=en.

171. Marjorie Dannenfelser, "The Suffragettes Would Not Agree With Feminists Today on Abortion," *Time*, November 24, 2015, https://time.com/4093214/suffragettes-abortion/.

172. Ibid.

173. Marjorie Dannenfelser, "Pro-Life Feminists Are Old-School," *National Review*, January 20, 2017, https://www.nationalreview.com/2017/01/snl-susan-b-anthony-early-feminists-opposed-abortion/.

174. "Dr. Elizabeth Blackwell," Feminists for Life of America, https://www.feministsforlife.org/herstory-dr-elizabeth-blackwell/.

NOTES

175. Michael W. McConnell, "How Not to Promote Serious Deliberation About Abortion," *University of Chicago Law Review* 58 (1991): 1188.

176. William Shakespeare, "Measure for Measure," Act 2, Scene 2 (Norwalk, Connecticut: Easton Press, 1992), 29.

177. Charlotte Alter, "Here's Why This Woman Filmed Her Own Abortion," *Time*, May 7, 2014, https://time.com/90860/abortion-emily-letts/.

178. Heather Wood Rudulph, "Why I Filmed My Abortion," *Cosmopolitan*, May 5, 2014, https://www.cosmopolitan.com/politics/a6674/why-i-filmed-my-abortion/.

179. Christine Sisto, "I Still Want to See an Abortion Video," *National Review*, May 13, 2014, https://www.nationalreview.com/2014/05/i-still-want-see-abortion-video-christine-sisto/.

180. William Shakespeare, Macbeth, Act 5, Scene 1 (Norwalk, Connecticut: Easton Press, 1992), 72.

181. Catharine MacKinnon, "*Roe v. Wade*: A Study in Male Ideology," in *Abortion: Moral and Legal Perspectives*, ed. J. Garfield and P. Hennessey (Amherst: University of Massachusetts Press, 1984).

182. Liz Plank (@feministabulous), Twitter, May 15, 2019, https://twitter.com/feministabulous/status/1128822738318237697?s=11.

183. Robyn Merrett, "Indiana Teen Who Fatally Stabbed Pregnant Cheerleader Girlfriend Sentenced to 65 Years Behind Bars," *People*, January 9, 2020, https://people.com/crime/indiana-teen-who-killed-pregnant-cheerleader-girlfriend-sentenced-65-years/.

184. Obianuju Ekeocha (@obianuju), Twitter, January 20, 2020, https://twitter.com/obianuju/status/1219195489859637249?s=11.

185. F. Scott Fitzgerald, "The Great Gatsby" (New York: Simon and Schuster, 1995), 187–188.

186. Sean Fitzpatrick, "Marching for Life, Mother Teresa, and Mrs. Clinton," *Crisis Magazine*, January 20, 2016, https://www.crisismagazine.com/2016/marching-for-life-mother-teresa-and-mrs-clinton.

187. Kylie Jenner, "To Our Daughter," *YouTube*, February 4, 2018, https://www.youtube.com/watch?v=BhIEIO0vaBE.

188. Carly Hoilman, "Listen to Your Heart, Not Hollywood Lesson From Kylie Jenner," *Catholic Vote*, March 16, 2018, https://catholicvote.org/listen-to-your-heart-not-hollywood-a-lesson-from-kylie-jenner/.

189. Cory Stieg, "This Is Kylie Jenner's Best Parenting Advice," *Refinery* 29, August 29, 2019, https://www.refinery29.com/en-us/2019/08/239569/kylie-jenner-parenting-advice-stormi.

190. Randy Alcorn, cited by Kathy Norquist and Stephanie Anderson, "Teens Who Choose Life in Unplanned Pregnancies Need Support and Respect, Not Shame," *Eternal Perspective Ministries*, June, 21, 2017, https://www.epm.org/blog/2017/Jun/21/teens-pregnancy-unsupport.

191. The Margaret Sanger Papers Project, "Birth Control or Race Control? Sanger and the Negro Project," New York University, *Fall* 2001, https://www.nyu.edu/projects/sanger/articles/bc_or_race_control.php.

192. "Planned Parenthood Honors King Herod With Lifetime Achievement Award," *Babylon Bee*, December 12, 2019, https://babylonbee.com/news/planned-parenthood-honors-king-herod-with-lifetime-achievement-award.

193. "Who We Are," *Planned Parenthood*, https://www.plannedparenthood.org/about-us/who-we-are.

NOTES

194. Kara Nesvig, "Miley Cyrus and Marc Jacobs Designed a Pink Hoodie That Benefits Planned Parenthood," *Teen Vogue*, June 5, 2019, https://www.teenvogue.com/story/miley-cyrus-and-marc-jacobs-designed-a-pink-hoodie-that-benefits-planned-parenthood.

195. Rose Minutaglio, "Miley Cyrus And Marc Jacobs Debut A 'Don't F*Ck With My Freedom' Hoodie Benefitting Planned Parenthood," June 4, 2019, https://www.elle.com/culture/celebrities/a27725846/miley-cyrus-marc-jacobs-hoodie-planned-parenthood/.

196. Katie Yoder, "Miley Cyrus Tells Jimmy Fallon: I'm a "Good Face" For Abortion and Planned Parenthood," *Life News*, May 19, 2016, https://www.lifenews.com/2016/05/19/miley-cyrus-tells-jimmy-fallon-im-a-good-face-for-abortion-and-planned-parenthood/.

197. "LIZZO, Billie Eilish, Ariana Grande, Lady Gaga, Halsey, John Legend, Nicki Minaj, Demi Lovato, Dua Lipa, G-Eazy, HAIM, Sara Bareilles, Troye Sivan, Macklemore, Megan Thee Stallion, Miley Cyrus, Kacey Musgraves, Carole King, Hayley Kiyoko, Bon Iver, Beck, Selena Gomez, and More Speak Out Against Abortion Restrictions," *Planned Parenthood*, August 26, 2019, https://www.plannedparenthood.org/about-us/newsroom/press-releases/lizzo-billie-eilish-ariana-grande-lady-gaga-halsey-john-legend-nicki-minaj-demi-lovato-beck-g-eazy-haim-sara-bareilles-troye-sivan-macklemore-megan-thee-stallion-miley-cyrus-kacey-musgraves-carole-king-hayley-kiyoko-bon-iver-dua-lipa-and-more-speak-out-against-abortion-restrictions.

198. Hannah Yasharoff, "Ariana Grande donates $250,000 from Atlanta concert to Planned Parenthood," *USA Today*, June 12, 2019, https://www.usatoday.com/story/life/people/2019/06/12/ariana-grande-donates-georgia-concert-money-planned-parenthood/1430405001/.

199. "It's time for companies to stand up for reproductive healthcare," Don't Ban Equality, https://dontbanequality.com/.

200. Sam Dorman, "Elizabeth Warren says she'll wear Planned Parenthood scarf to her inauguration," December 3, 2019, https://www.foxnews.com/politics/elizabeth-warren-planned-parenthood-inauguration.

201. Ibid.

202. Ema O'Connor, "Planned Parenthood's New President Wants To Focus On Non-abortion Health Care," *BuzzFeed News*, January 7, 2019, https://www.buzzfeednews.com/article/emaoconnor/planned-parenthood-leana-wen-health-care-abortion-politics?utm_source=dynamic&utm_campaign=bffbbuzzfeed&ref=bffbbuzzfeed.

203. Glenn Kessler, "Fact Checker," *Washington Post*, January 7, 2019, https://www.washingtonpost.com/politics/2019/01/07/about-fact-checker/.

204. "We Are Planned Parenthood," *Planned Parenthood*, https://www.plannedparenthood.org/uploads/filer_public/2e/da/2eda3f50-82aa-4ddb-acce-c2854c4ea80b/2018-2019_annual_report.pdf.

205. "2017–2018 Annual Report," *Planned Parenthood*, https://www.plannedparenthood.org/uploads/filer_public/80/d7/80d7d7c7-977c-4036-9c61-b3801741b441/190118-annualreport18-p01.pdf.

206. "Induced Abortion in the United States," *Guttmacher Institute*, September, 2019, https://www.guttmacher.org/fact-sheet/induced-abortion-united-states.

207. "U.S. Abortion Statistics: Facts and figures relating to the frequency of abortion in the United States," Abort73.com, https://abort73.com/abortion_facts/us_abortion_statistics/.

208. Carole Novielli, "Though U.S. abortions have dropped, Planned Parenthood now does 40% of them," *Live Action*, September 19, 2019, https://www.liveaction.org/news/planned-parenthood-almost-40-percent-us-abortions/.

209. "Get Care," *Planned Parenthood*, https://www.plannedparenthood.org/get-care.

NOTES

210. Mollie Hemingway, "FACT CHECK: The Largest Women's Health Care Provider In America Is NOT Planned Parenthood," *The Federalist*, August 3, 2015, https://thefederalist.com/2015/08/03/fact-check-the-largest-womens-health-care-provider-in-america-is-not-planned-parenthood/.

211. Melissa Barnhart, "7 states already allow abortion up to birth—not just New York," January 30, 2019, https://www.christianpost.com/news/7-states-already-allow-abortion-up-to-birth-not-just-new-york.html.

212. Kate Bryan, "Planned Parenthood "Lamborghini" Exec Haggles Again Over Baby Parts Prices In New Video," *Center for Medical Progress*, April 26, 2017, http://www.centerformedicalprogress.org/2017/04/2027/.

213. David Daleiden, "Second Planned Parenthood Senior Executive Haggles Over Baby Parts Prices, Changes Abortion Methods," *Center for Medical Progress*, July 21, 2015, http://www.centerformedicalprogress.org/2015/07/second-planned-parenthood-senior-executive-haggles-over-baby-parts-prices-changes-abortion-methods/.

214. Maureen Collins, "Planned Parenthood Staffers Jokingly Called the Freezer Containing Aborted Baby Parts 'The Nursery,'" *Life News*, August 8, 2017, https://www.lifenews.com/2017/08/08/planned-parenthood-staffers-jokingly-called-the-freezer-containing-aborted-baby-parts-the-nursery/.

215. Planned Parenthood (@PPFA), Twitter, Mar 10, 2020, 10:55 a.m., https://twitter.com/PPFA/status/1237436827813937153.

216. Planned Parenthood Gulf Coast, "National Day of Appreciation for Abortion Providers," *Planned Parenthood Website*, March 8, 2019, https://www.plannedparenthood.org/planned-parenthood-gulf-coast/blog/national-day-of-appreciation-for-abortion-providers.

217. Press Release, "CMS Releases Recommendations on Adult Elective Surgeries, Non-Essential Medical, Surgical, and Dental Procedures During COVID-19 Response," March 18, 2020, https://www.cms.gov/newsroom/press-releases/cms-releases-recommendations-adult-elective-surgeries-non-essential-medical-surgical-and-dental.

218. Kate Smith, "Abortion in Ohio will continue, despite Attorney General order to stop," *CBS News*, March 22, 2020, https://www.cbsnews.com/news/abortion-in-ohio-will-continue-despite-attorney-general-order-to-stop/.

219. Steven Ertelt, "Ohio Abortion Clinics Ordered to Stop Killing Babies: Abortions are Not "Essential" Procedures," *Life News*, March 21, 2020, https://www.lifenews.com/2020/03/21/ohio-abortion-clinics-ordered-to-close-abortions-are-not-essential-surgical-procedures/.

220. Micaiah Bilger, "Planned Parenthood Closes Some Centers, Keeps Abortion Clinics Open Because Women 'Need' to Kill Their Babies," *Life News*, March 20, 2020, https://www.lifenews.com/2020/03/20/planned-parenthood-stops-legitimate-health-care-but-will-kill-babies-because-women-need-abortions/.

221. Planned Parenthood, "Donald Trump, President of the United States," *Planned Parenthood Website*, https://www.plannedparenthoodaction.org/tracking-trump/player/donald-trump.

222. Planned Parenthood Action (@PPact), Twitter, March 15, 2020, https://twitter.com/ppact/status/1239371385044156417?s=11.

223. Kate Smith, "Planned Parenthood launches $45 million investment in 2020 elections," *CBS News*, January 6, 2020, https://www.cbsnews.com/news/planned-parenthood-45-million-we-decide-2020-elections-investment-today/.

224. "Contributions to Federal Candidates, 2020 cycle," OpenSecrets.org, https://www.opensecrets.org/pacs/pacgot.php?cmte=C00314617.

NOTES

225. "We Are Planned Parenthood," *Planned Parenthood*, https://www.plannedparent hood.org/uploads/filer_public/2e/da/2eda3f50-82aa-4ddb-acce-c2854c4ea80b/2018-2019 _annual_report.pdf.

226. "We Are Planned Parenthood," *Planned Parenthood*.

227. Dr. Susan Berry, "Trump Administration Enacts Rule Ending Family Planning Funds to Abortion Providers," *Breitbart*, July 17, 2019, https://www.breitbart.com/politics /2019/07/17/trump-administration-enacts-rule-ending-family-planning-funds-to-abortion -providers/.

228. Adam Liptak, "Supreme Court Lets Kentucky Abortion Ultrasound Law Take Effect," *New York Times*, https://www.nytimes.com/2019/12/09/us/supreme-court-ken tucky-abortion-ultrasound.html?login=smartlock&auth=login-smartlock&login=smart lock&auth=login-smartlock.

229. Adam Liptak, "Supreme Court Lets Kentucky Abortion Ultrasound Law Take Effect."

230. Mollie Hemingway, "FACT CHECK: The Largest Women's Health Care Provider In America Is NOT Planned Parenthood."

231. Alexandra DeSanctis, "Planned Parenthood's New Annual Report Disproves Its Own Narrative," *National Review*, January 21, 2019, https://www.nationalreview .com/2019/01/planned-parenthood-annual-report-disproves-narrative/.

232. *Box v. Planned Parenthood of Indiana and Kentucky*, 587 U.S._ (2019), 18.

233. Mara Hvistendahl, *Unnatural Selection: Choosing Boys Over Girls, and the Conse-quences of a World Full of Men* (New York: Public Affairs, 2011), 5–6.

234. "Marketplace," *Planned Parenthood*, https://marketplace.plannedparenthood.org/.

235. Margaret Sanger, "My Way to Peace," *The Public Papers of Margaret Sanger*, https:// www.nyu.edu/projects/sanger/webedition/app/documents/show.php?sangerDoc=129037 .xml.

236. Ian Tuttle, "What Ben Carson Knows about Planned Parenthood," *National Review*, August 14, 2015, https://www.nationalreview.com/2015/08/planned-parenthood -ben-carson/.

237. Ian Tuttle, "What Ben Carson Knows about Planned Parenthood."

238. The Margaret Sanger Papers Project, "Birth Control or Race Control? Sanger and the Negro Project."

239. Ibid.

240. John J. Conley, S.J., "Margaret Sanger was a eugenicist. Why are we still celebrat-ing her?" *America, The Jesuit Review*, November 27, 2017, https://www.americamagazine.org /politics-society/2017/11/27/margaret-sanger-was-eugenicist-why-are-we-still-celebrating-her.

241. Margaret Sanger, *Margaret Sanger: An Autobiography* (New York: W. W. Norton, 1938), 366–367.

242. The Margaret Sanger Papers Project, "Birth Control or Race Control? Sanger and the Negro Project."

243. "Our History," *Planned Parenthood*, https://www.plannedparenthood.org/about-us /who-we-are/our-history.

244. Diane Paul, *Controlling Human Heredity: 1865–Present*, quoted in *Box v. Planned Parenthood of Indiana and Kentucky*, 587 U.S. ___ (2019), 14, https://www.supremecourt.gov /opinions/18pdf/18-483_3d9g.pdf.

245. *Box v. Planned Parenthood of Indiana and Kentucky*, 587 U.S._ (2019).

246. A. Guttmacher, *Babies By Choice or By Chance*, quoted in *Box v. Planned Parenthood of Indiana and Kentucky*, 14, https://www.supremecourt.gov/opinions/18pdf/18-483_3d9g .pdf.

NOTES

247. Ibid.

248. "Planned Parenthood Exploits Martin Luther King to Promote Abortion, Attacks Alveda King," *Life News*, January 22, 2019, https://www.lifenews.com/2019/01/22 /planned-parenthood-exploits-martin-luther-king-to-promote-abortion-attacks-alveda-king/.

249. New York State Department of Health, "Table 23: Induced Abortion and Abortion Ratios by Race/Ethnicity and Resident County New York State – 2016," https://health.ny.gov/ statistics/vital_statistics/2016/table23.htm.

250. "Planned Parenthood & Racism," *Students for Life of America*, https://studentsforlife .org/planned-parenthood-racism/.

251. Lifesite News, "One Quarter of Blacks Missing from Abortion Genocide Says Dr. Alveda King," *Catholic Exchange*, August 25, 2007, https://catholicexchange.com /one-quarter-of-blacks-missing-from-abortion-genocide-says-dr-alveda-king.

252. Dr. Jerry Newcombe, "Dr. Alveda King Interview: Planned Parenthood Targeting Blacks?" *American Family Association*, January 24, 2019, https://www.afa.net/the-stand /culture/2019/01/dr-alveda-king-interview-planned-parenthood-targeting-blacks/.

253. Ian Tuttle, "What Ben Carson Knows about Planned Parenthood."

254. "10 Celebrities Who Are Speaking Out Against Abortion," *Save the Storks*, September 8, 2017, https://savethestorks.com/2017/09/10-celebrities-speaking-abortion/.

255. *Box v. Planned Parenthood of Indiana and Kentucky*, 587 U.S._ (2019), 18.

256. Jonah Goldberg, "A Dark Past," *National Review*, June 24, 2008, https://www .nationalreview.com/2008/06/dark-past-jonah-goldberg/.

257. Ibid.

258. "In Defense of Margaret Sanger on Eugenics," *Wall Street Journal Opinion*, September 15, 2019, https://www.wsj.com/articles/in-defense-of-margaret-sanger-on-eugenics -11568554915.

259. Mona Charen, "Mrs. Clinton Can't Defend Patron Saint of Planned Parenthood," *National Review*, April 24, 2009, https://www.nationalreview.com/2009/04/mrs -clinton-cant-defend-patron-saint-planned-parenthood-mona-charen/.

260. Ibid.

261. Christopher Hitchens, "A Left-Wing Atheist's Case Against Abortion," *Crisis Magazine*, December 5, 2019, https://www.crisismagazine.com/2019/a-left-wing-atheists-case -against-abortion.

262. Liz Hayes, "WALL OF SEPARATION BLOG: Abortion Is A Church-State Separation Issue. That's Why We Need To Stop The Bans," *Americans United for Separation of Church and State*, May 22, 2019, https://www.au.org/blogs/wall-of-separation/abortion -is-a-church-state-separation-issue-thats-why-we-need-to-stop-the.

263. "Who We Are," *Americans United for Separation of Church and State*, https://www.au .org/who-we-are.

264. "SEPTEMBER 15, 1982, REAGAN QUOTES AND SPEECHES," *Ronald Reagan Presidential Foundation and Institute*, https://www.reaganfoundation.org/ronald-reagan /reagan-quotes-speeches/radio-address-to-the-nation-on-prayer/.

265. Christopher Hitchens, "A Left-Wing Atheist's Case Against Abortion."

266. "Billy Graham Will Not Be Advisor to Obama Because of His Abortion Position," *Christian Coalition*, http://www.cc.org/news/billy_graham_will_not_be_advisor_obama_because _his_abortion_position?_cf_chl_jschl_tk__=eb3dcce8be2defa69fc5d705f0a36f97d3ad de8c-1596054984-0-Af3uMFcfhzkhstVL1m6puiJc-DAJFtdsdh5_PfoJQc3JbNWZTvS0b1X t2N_54qCvlKsXPMcwgSnJA5GRU1Dl0eE6QpzaD5jtObCkWaUpOGRtATuifmw608jTHHV vEY-9qTLS34V_NjgU1Mtn8cYg1IV_iB1WvBQu4XzvECRLBTtMJwIoNX4hyreEkvqxNf3gX7B

NOTES

kHx8-y5a0eVW5HHvDz_CqTeUIH1IdTghXm-N-qkpaAnMOg_pXMxsaRIhlO28zNbqo
jFtVQ7esZS7eQc6qmGoMp3XsgylyZloZFnXwg21YNMO3yDUg6KEi2hBUQFDeJVfoTyFba4
-DDRy5Lq660F-RJ1XlXaga5HN39AQPEUdFPB5qx_7jIU4tCl_nqif0eQ.

267. Aleksandr I. Solzhenitsyn, *The Gulag Archipelago, 1918–1956: An Experiment in Literary Investigation*, V–VII.

268. Martin Luther King Jr., cited by Bob Herbert, "The Lost Voice of Protest," *New York Times*, January 18, 2007, https://www.nytimes.com/2007/01/18/opinion/18herbert.html.

269. Adrienne Lafrance, "Clinton's Unapologetic Defense of Abortion Rights," *The Atlantic*, October 20, 2016, https://www.theatlantic.com/health/archive/2016/10/hillary-clintons-powerful-defense-of-abortion-rights/504866/.

270. "October 11, 1984 Debate Transcript," *The Commission on Presidential Debates*, https://www.debates.org/voter-education/debate-transcripts/october-11-1984-debate-transcript/.

271. "Quotes on Argument," *The Samuel Johnson Sound Bite Page*, https://www.samueljohnson.com/argument.html.

272. The Rubin Report, "Trump, Trans, Religion, Abortion, and Tax Cuts | Ben Shapiro | POLITICS | Rubin Report," *YouTube*, https://www.youtube.com/watch?v=s9Iwamztdq A&t=4193s.

273. Frederica Mathewes-Green, "When Abortion Suddenly Stopped Making Sense," *National Review*, January 22, 2016, https://www.nationalreview.com/2016/01/abortion-roe-v-wade-unborn-children-women-feminism-march-life/.

274. "How Many Couples are Waiting to Adopt?" *American Adoptions*, https://www.americanadoptions.com/pregnant/waiting_adoptive_families.

275. Ibid.

276. Senator Dianne Feinstein (@SenFeinstein), Twitter, January 22, 2020, https://twitter.com/senfeinstein/status/1219990253370531844?s=11.

277. Rachel Jones, PhD, Jenna Jerman, MPH, Meghan Ingerick, BA, "Which Abortion Patients Have Had a Prior Abortion? Findings from the 2014 U.S. Abortion Patient Survey," *Journal of Women's Health*, January 1, 2018, https://www.ncbi.nlm.nih.gov/pmc/articles/PMC5771530/.

278. Clarke D. Forsythe, *Abuse of Discretion: Inside the Story of* Roe v. Wade (New York: Encounter Books, 2013), 320.

279. Gertrude Himmelfarb, *The Demoralization of Society: From Victorian Virtues to Modern Values* (New York: Vintage Books, 1994), 248.

280. "If Abortion is Made Illegal, Women Will Die in Back Alleys," *Catholic News Agency*, https://www.catholicnewsagency.com/resources/apologetics/defending-life/if-abortion-is-made-illegal-women-will-die-in-back-alleys.

281. Bernard Nathanson, *"Aborting America: A Doctor's Personal Report on the Agonizing Issue of Abortion"* (Ontario, Canada: Life Cycle Books, 1979).

282. Young America's Foundation, "Legalizing abortion doesn't make it safe ft. Kristan Hawkins, #TruthStraightUp," *YouTube*, January 24, 2020, https://www.youtube.com/watch?v=j23P7fnLLRY&feature=youtu.be.

283. "7 Effective and Risk-free Home Remedies for Abortion," *Hub Culture*, https://hubculture.com/hubs/855/news/884/.

284. Inga Muscio, *Cunt: A Declaration of Independence* (New York: Hachette Book Group, 2018), 53.

285. Ibid., 54.

286. Ibid., 55

287. Massachusetts Down Syndrome Congress, "Frank Stephens' POWERFUL Speech on Down Syndrome," *YouTube*, October 30, 2017, https://www.youtube.com /watch?v=vtS91Jd5mac.

288. Roy B. Sessions M.D., "More on the Pregnant Cancer Patient: To Terminate or No," July 17, 2016, https://www.psychologytoday.com/intl/blog/the-cancer-experience/201607 /more-the-pregnant-cancer-patient-terminate-or-no.

289. William Hemsworth, "Understanding the Principle of Double Effect to do the Most Good," *Patheos*, January 29, 2020, https://www.patheos.com/blogs /thepursuitofholiness/2020/01/principle-of-double-effect/.

290. Catherine Larmon, "Ireland Abortion is not the Answer," *Praying Through the Scriptures*, September 29, 2014, https://spiritualfoodforthesoul.wordpress.com/2014/09/29 /ireland-abortion-is-not-the-answer/.

291. ABC News, "Tim Tebow Interview Exclusive on Girlfriends, Taylor Swift, His Foundation and the New York Jets," *YouTube*, April 13, 2012, https://www.youtube.com /watch?v=B9NzIoaB45I.

292. "Ectopic Pregnancy," *Mayo Clinic*, https://www.mayoclinic.org/diseases-conditions /ectopic-pregnancy/symptoms-causes/syc-20372088.

293. Ibid.

294. Bill Fortenberry, "Fact Sheet on Ectopic Pregnancy," *The Personhood Initiative*, http://www.personhoodinitiative.com/fact-sheet-on-ectopic-pregnancy.html.

295. Dr. Patrick Johnston, "Does an ectopic pregnancy justify intentionally killing the baby?" *Celebrate Life Magazine*, 2016 Winter, https://www.clmagazine.org/topic/medicine-science /does-an-ectopic-pregnancy-justify-intentionally-killing-the-baby/.

296. Paul Sims, Jill Foster, "The mother who risked everything to have her ectopic baby," *Daily Mail*, June 26, 2011, https://www.dailymail.co.uk/health/article-2008476/The -mother-risked-ectopic-baby.html.

297. Katie Moisse, "Baby Born Deformed After Misdiagnosed Ectopic Pregnancy," *ABC News*, January 23, 2012, https://abcnews.go.com/Health/w_ParentingResource /baby-born-deformed-misdiagnosed-ectopic-pregnancy/story?id=15421441.

298. Ibid.

299. "Everything you need to know about preeclampsia," *Medical News Today*, https:// www.medicalnewstoday.com/articles/252025.

300. "PREECLAMPSIA," *March of Dimes*, https://www.marchofdimes.org/complications /preeclampsia.aspx.

301. Sharon Mazel, "What Happens If You Get an Ovarian Cyst When You're Pregnant?" *What To Expect*, May 12, 2020, https://www.whattoexpect.com/pregnancy/your-health /ovarian-cysts-during-pregnancy/.

302. "What is a high-risk pregnancy?" *National Institutes of Health* (NIH), https://www .nichd.nih.gov/health/topics/pregnancy/conditioninfo/high-risk.

303. "HIV/AIDS and Pregnancy," *MedlinePlus*, https://medlineplus.gov/hivaidsand pregnancy.html.

304. "Reasons U.S. Women Have Abortions," *Guttmacher*, https://www.guttmacher.org /sites/default/files/pdfs/tables/370305/3711005t3.pdf.

305. "10 Celebrities Who Are Speaking Out Against Abortion," *Save the Storks*.

306. "Martin Sheen reveals wife was conceived in rape, talks about strong anti-abortion views," *Metro Voice*, November 6, 2013, https://metrovoicenews.com/martin-sheen-reveals -wife-was-conceived-in-rape-talks-about-strong-anti-abortion-views/.

NOTES

307. Live Science Staff, "What's the Youngest Age at Which a Woman Can Give Birth?" *Live Science*, March 30, 2011, https://www.livescience.com/33170-youngest-age-give-birth -pregnancy.html.

308. "U.S. Abortion Statistics," *Abort73*, https://abort73.com/abortion_facts/us_abortion _statistics/.

309. Fondation Jérôme Lejeune, "I AM A MAN WITH DOWN SYNDROME AND MY LIFE IS WORTH LIVING. Frank Stephens' speech at the UN," *YouTube*, March 18, 2018, https://www.youtube.com/watch?v=1d8ocuPrlT8&t=337s.

310. Massachusetts Down Syndrome Congress, "Frank Stephens' POWERFUL Speech on Down Syndrome," *YouTube*, October 30, 2017, https://www.youtube.com /watch?v=vtS91Jd5mac.

311. Huckabee, "Why Abortion Is Based On The Logic Of Slavery," *YouTube*, January 20, 2018, https://www.youtube.com/watch?v=HrKw33o41ag.

312. Marilyn Monroe, "The Magic of Marilyn Monroe," *House and Garden*, https://www .houseandgarden.co.uk/gallery/marilyn-monroe-quotes-pictures.

313. "Breaker Morant," 1980, *IMDB*, https://www.imdb.com/title/tt0080310/.

314. "Testimony from Nurse Jill L. Stanek during the Born Alive Infant Protection Act Congressional Hearings," *California ProLife Council*, https://www.californiaprolife .org/testimony-from-nurse-jill-l-stanek-during-the-born-alive-infant-protection-act -congressional-hearings/.

315. David Stout, "Abortion Rights Advocate Says He Lied About Procedure," *New York Times*, February 26, 1997, https://www.nytimes.com/1997/02/26/us/an-abortion-rights -advocate-says-he-lied-about-procedure.html.

316. Ibid.

317. Lawrence B. Finer, Stanley K. Henshaw, "Abortion Incidence and Services In the United States in 2000," *Guttmacher*, https://www.guttmacher.org/sites/default/files/pdfs /pubs/psrh/full/3500603.pdf.

318. H.R. 2175 – Born Alive Infants Protection Act, 2002, https://www.congress.gov /bill/107th-congress/house-bill/2175/text.

319. "Testimony from Nurse Jill L. Stanek during the Born Alive Infant Protection Act Congressional Hearings," *California ProLife Council*, https://www.californiaprolife.org /testimony-from-nurse-jill-l-stanek-during-the-born-alive-infant-protection-act-congressional -hearings/.

320. Chris Smith, "Baby Born Alive at 23 Weeks Was Gasping for Air. Abortion Clinic Put Baby in a Bag, Threw Her in the Trash," *Life News*, September 13, 2019, https://www .lifenews.com/2019/09/13/baby-born-alive-at-23-weeks-was-gasping-for-air-abortion-clinic -put-baby-in-a-bag-threw-her-in-the-trash/.

321. Jennifer Johnson, "One of the best Pro-life speeches EVER! Gianna Jessen abor- tion survivor Full video," *YouTube*, https://www.youtube.com/watch?v=hOWMmx6eBjU.

322. Adam Eley, Jo Adnitt, "The failed abortion survivor whose mum thought she was dead," June 5, 2018, https://www.bbc.com/news/health-44357373.

323. "They Are Real: Meet Born-Alive Abortion Survivors," *Human Defense*, March 4, 2019, https://humandefense.com/meet-born-alive-abortion-survivors/.

324. Ibid.

325. Tim Pearce, "'They chose life': GOP congressman tells story of how his staffer was almost aborted," *Washington Examiner*, November 14, 2019, https://www.washingtonexaminer .com/news/they-chose-life-gop-congressman-tells-story-of-how-his-staffer-was-almost -aborted.

326. Götz Aly, *Hitler's Beneficiaries: Plunder, Racial War, and The Nazi Welfare State* (New York: Henry Hold and Company, 2006).

327. *Box v. Planned Parenthood of Indiana and Kentucky*, 587 U.S._ (2019), 18.

328. Diana Schaub, "A hidden cause of Baltimore's population loss: abortion," *Baltimore Sun*, January 23, 2012, https://www.baltimoresun.com/opinion/op-ed/bs-ed-abortion-population-20120123-8-story.html.

329. David Buer, "Steve Jobs and the March for Life," *Deseret News*, February 2, 2017, https://www.deseret.com/2017/2/2/20605332/steve-jobs-and-the-march-for-life.

330. "Remarks by President Trump at the 47th Annual March for Life," *WhiteHouse.gov*, January 24, 2020, https://www.whitehouse.gov/briefings-statements/remarks-president-trump-47th-annual-march-life/.

331. Mother Teresa, cited by Josephen Pronechen, "What if Pro Life Saints Join the March for Life?" *National Catholic Register*, January 19, 2018, https://www.ncregister.com/blog/joseph-pronechen/what-if-pro-life-saints-join-the-march-for-life.

332. Tom McKay, "Here's Why George Carlin's 1996 Rant on Pro-Life Conservatives Still Rings True," *Mic*, December 2, 2015, https://www.mic.com/articles/129542/here-s-why-george-carlin-s-1996-rant-on-pro-life-conservatives-still-rings-true.

333. Mohammad Fazel Zarandi, Jonathan S. Feinstein, Edward H. Kaplan, "Yale Study Finds Twice as Many Undocumented Immigrants as Previous Estimates," *Yale Insights*, September 21, 2018, https://insights.som.yale.edu/insights/yale-study-finds-twice-as-many-undocumented-immigrants-as-previous-estimates.

334. "Number of Abortions – Abortion Counters," http://www.numberofabortions.com/.

335. "Services," *Metroplex Women's Clinic*, https://www.metroplexwomensclinic.com/services/.

336. "Pregnancy Centers," *Vitae Foundation*, https://vitaefoundation.org/pregcenters.

337. Dinesh D'Souza, *Ronald Reagan: How an Ordinary Man Became an Extraordinary Leader* (New York: Free Press, 1997), 208.

338. Fred Schruers, "Jack Nicholson: The Rolling Stone Interview," *Rolling Stone*, August 14, 1986, https://www.rollingstone.com/culture/culture-features/jack-nicholson-the-rolling-stone-interview-69393/.

339. Michael W. Chapman, "Jack Nicholson on Abortion: 'I'm Positively Against It' – 'I Never Would Have Gotten to Live,'" *CNS News*, September 4, 2013, https://www.cnsnews.com/news/article/michael-w-chapman/jack-nicholson-abortion-i-m-positively-against-it-i-never-would-have.

340. Lesli White, "6 Celebrities Who Are Openly Pro-Life," *Belief Net*, https://www.beliefnet.com/entertainment/celebrities/6-celebrities-who-are-openly-pro-life.aspx.

341. Associated Press, "Justin Bieber's mom, Pattie Mallette, lays bare her painful past and turns to God in new book," *Fox News*, September 24, 2012 (Updated April 6, 2016), https://www.foxnews.com/entertainment/justin-biebers-mom-pattie-mallette-lays-bare-her-painful-past-and-turns-to-god-in-new-book.

342. "Justin Bieber Takes Mom to Hillsong Church After Years of Estrangement," *CBN News*, January 28, 2018, https://www1.cbn.com/cbnnews/entertainment/2018/january/justin-bieber-takes-mom-to-hillsong-church-after-years-of-estrangement.

343. Abraham Lincoln, speech to Fourteenth Indiana Regiment, March 17, 1865, https://www.nps.gov/libo/learn/historyculture/thoughts-on-slavery.htm.

344. Ayn Rand, "Atlas Shrugged," https://princetonlibrary.bibliocommons.com/item/quotation/1330117057

345. Jonah Goldberg, "Liberal theory of justice doesn't support abortion," *Chicago Tribune*, July 21, 2015, https://www.chicagotribune.com/opinion/commentary/ct-planned -parenthood-liberals-abortion-goldberg-20150721-column.html.

346. John Rawls, "The University of Chicago Law Review," *The University of Chicago*, Summer 1997, https://chicagounbound.uchicago.edu/cgi/viewcontent.cgi?article=5633&context =uclrev.

347. John Rawls, *A Theory of Justice* (Cambridge, MA: Belknap Press of Harvard University Press, 1971), 12.

348. John Milton, *Paradise Lost* (New York: Barnes and Noble Classics, 2004), 54.

349. Nigel Jones, "From Stalin to Hitler, the most murderous regimes in the world," *Mail Online*, October 7, 2014, https://www.dailymail.co.uk/home/moslive/article-2091670 /Hitler-Stalin-The-murderous-regimes-world.html.

350. John Hirschauer, "Pro-Life Amicus Brief Reveals the Mendacity of the Pro-Choice Movement," *National Review*, January 10, 2020, https://www.nationalreview.com/2020/01 /pro-life-amicus-brief-reveals-the-mendacity-of-the-pro-choice-movement/.

INDEX

INDEX

INDEX

INDEX

INDEX

INDEX

INDEX

INDEX

INDEX

INDEX